Transform Your Gut Health

Quiet Your Gut, Boost Fiber Intake, and Reduce Inflammation with These Gut-Healthy Recipes

BY
ADEEL ANJUM

CONTENTS

INTRODUCTION

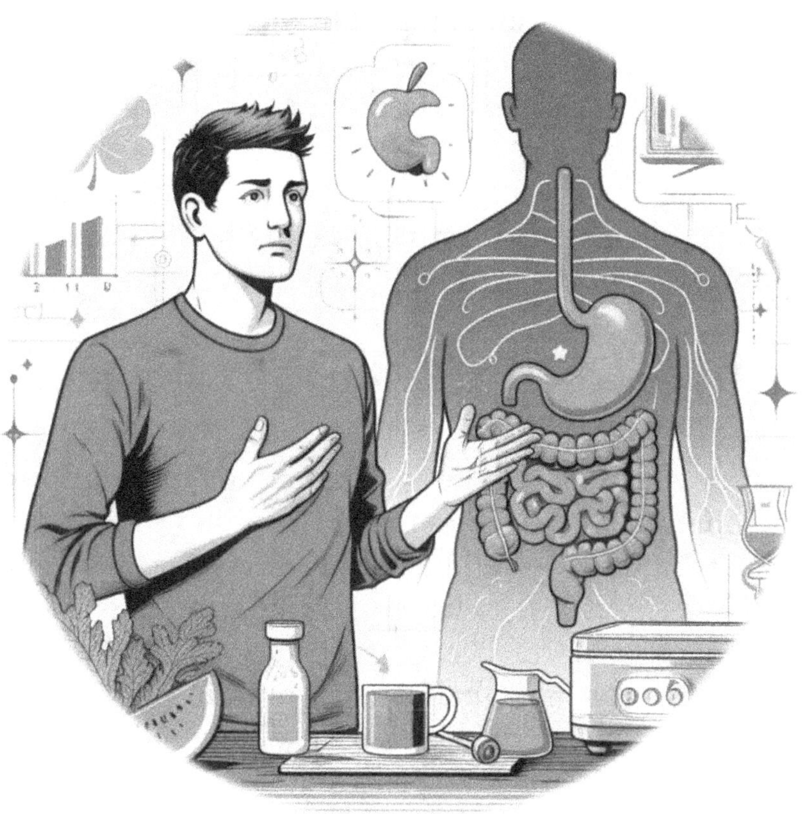

Gut health is a fundamental aspect of overall well-being, often overlooked in conventional healthcare. It encompasses the delicate balance of microorganisms residing in the gastrointestinal tract and plays a pivotal role in numerous bodily functions beyond digestion. Understanding the significance of gut health involves appreciating its multifaceted impact on physical, mental, and even emotional health.

At its core, the gastrointestinal tract serves as the body's primary interface with the external environment, tasked with the crucial responsibility of processing and assimilating nutrients while defending against harmful pathogens. Within this intricate ecosystem, a diverse array of microorganisms, collectively known as the gut microbiota, coexists in symbiosis with the human host. This dynamic relationship is crucial for maintaining homeostasis and optimal functioning throughout the body.

Overview of the Gut Microbiome

The gut microbiome, comprising trillions of microorganisms, represents a complex ecosystem unique to each individual. This diverse community includes bacteria, viruses, fungi, and archaea, collectively influencing various physiological processes, from metabolism and immune function to neurological signaling. The composition and diversity of the gut microbiome are influenced by numerous factors, including genetics, diet, lifestyle, and environmental exposures.

Research has revealed the profound implications of the gut microbiome on human health, highlighting its involvement in modulating immune responses, regulating metabolism, and even influencing cognitive function. A balanced and resilient gut microbiome is associated with enhanced resilience to disease and improved overall well-being. Conversely, disruptions in microbial equilibrium, known as dysbiosis, have been implicated in the pathogenesis of various health conditions, including inflammatory bowel diseases, metabolic disorders, and even mental health disorders.

How Diet Affects Gut Health

Diet stands as one of the most influential determinants of gut health, exerting a profound impact on the composition and activity of the gut microbiome. The dietary choices we make directly shape the microbial communities inhabiting our gastrointestinal tract, with far-reaching consequences for health and disease. Embracing a gut-friendly diet involves prioritizing whole, nutrient-dense foods while minimizing the consumption of processed, inflammatory-inducing fare.

Central to promoting gut health is the incorporation of dietary fiber, found abundantly in fruits, vegetables, whole grains, and legumes. Fiber serves as a vital substrate for beneficial gut bacteria, fueling their growth and metabolic activity. By fermenting fiber, these microbes produce short-chain fatty acids (SCFAs), which play a key role in maintaining gut barrier integrity, regulating immune function, and modulating inflammation.

Furthermore, fermented foods rich in probiotics, such as yogurt, kefir, sauerkraut, and kimchi, offer additional support for gut health by introducing live beneficial bacteria into the digestive tract. These probiotic-rich foods contribute to microbial diversity and may confer various health benefits, including enhanced digestion, immune modulation, and reduced risk of gastrointestinal disorders.

In contrast, diets high in refined sugars, saturated fats, and processed foods have been implicated in disrupting gut microbial balance and promoting inflammation. Excessive consumption of sugary beverages, refined carbohydrates, and artificial additives can fuel the proliferation of pathogenic bacteria while diminishing the abundance of beneficial microbes, predisposing individuals to gut dysbiosis and associated health complications.

Common Signs of Poor Gut Health

Recognizing the signs of poor gut health is essential for early intervention and targeted intervention strategies. While symptoms may vary among individuals, several common indicators suggest underlying gastrointestinal dysfunction and microbial imbalance. These signs encompass a spectrum of digestive disturbances, systemic manifestations, and even psychological symptoms, underscoring the interconnectedness of gut health with overall well-being.

Digestive issues, such as chronic bloating, abdominal discomfort, irregular bowel movements, and gastrointestinal distress, often signal underlying imbalances in the gut microbiome. These symptoms may arise from dysbiosis, impaired gut motility, or compromised intestinal barrier function, highlighting the intricate interplay between diet, lifestyle, and gut health.

Furthermore, systemic manifestations of poor gut health may manifest as unexplained weight fluctuations, persistent fatigue, or compromised immune function. Inadequate nutrient absorption, chronic inflammation, and immune dysregulation can contribute to metabolic disturbances, energy imbalances, and susceptibility to recurrent infections.

Skin conditions, including acne, eczema, and psoriasis, may also reflect underlying disruptions in gut health, with inflammation and immune dysregulation playing prominent roles in dermatological manifestations. Moreover, emerging research suggests a bidirectional relationship between the gut and the skin, implicating gut microbiota in modulating cutaneous immunity and inflammatory responses.

Autoimmune disorders, characterized by aberrant immune responses targeting self-tissues, often involve perturbations in gut microbial composition and intestinal barrier integrity. Dysregulated immune signaling, coupled with compromised gut barrier function, can facilitate the translocation of microbial antigens, triggering systemic inflammation and autoimmunity.

Introduction to the Concept of Gut-Healthy Recipes

Central to nurturing gut health is the integration of dietary strategies aimed at fostering microbial diversity, supporting gut barrier integrity, and modulating inflammation. Gut-healthy recipes serve as a cornerstone of this approach, providing practical, delicious, and nutritionally dense options to support optimal gastrointestinal function and overall well-being.

These recipes are thoughtfully crafted to incorporate ingredients rich in dietary fiber, prebiotics, probiotics, and anti-inflammatory compounds, thereby promoting a thriving gut ecosystem. From vibrant salads and hearty soups to wholesome main courses and delectable desserts, each recipe is designed to nourish the body while tantalizing the taste buds.

By embracing gut-healthy recipes as part of a holistic approach to wellness, individuals can empower themselves to take proactive steps toward optimizing gut health and cultivating vitality from within. Through mindful eating habits and culinary creativity, we can harness the transformative potential of food to fuel our journey toward vibrant health and well-being.

In the pages that follow, you will embark on a culinary adventure, exploring an array of flavorful and nutrient-rich recipes designed to invigorate your palate and invigorate your gut. Whether you're seeking hearty breakfast options, satisfying snacks, or wholesome meals, you'll find an abundance of inspiration to support your quest for optimal gut health.

Join us as we embark on a journey to transform your gut health, one delicious bite at a time. Together, we'll unlock the power of nutrition to nourish your body, elevate your mood, and cultivate lasting vitality. Get ready to savor the flavors of health and embark on a journey toward a happier, healthier you.

Part 1: Fundamentals of Gut Health

Chapter 01

The Gut Microbiome Explained

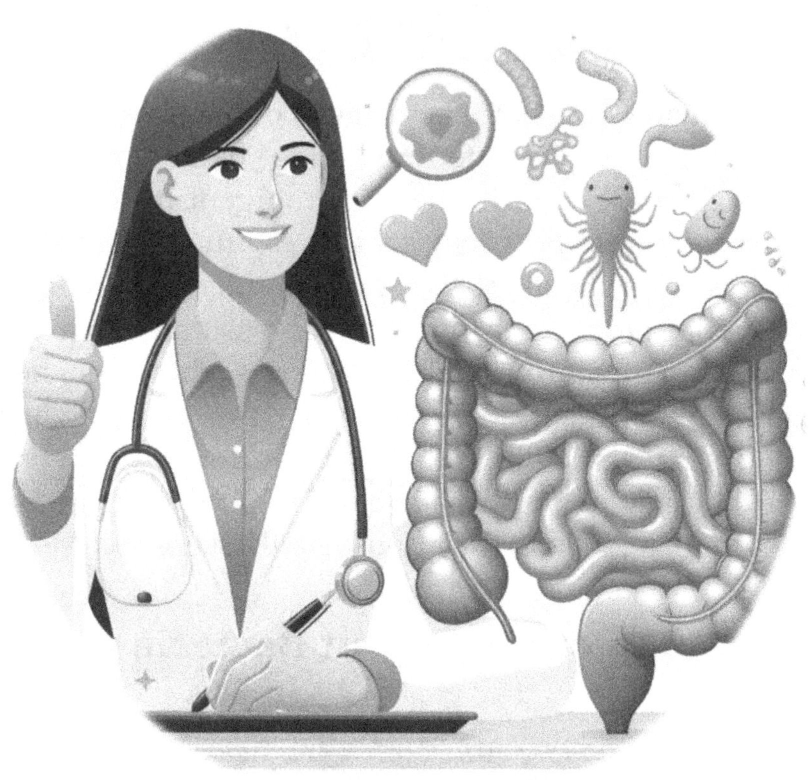

Definition of the Gut Microbiome

The gut microbiome is a vast and intricate community of microorganisms that reside in the human digestive tract. These microorganisms include bacteria, viruses, fungi, and archaea. Collectively, they perform essential functions that contribute to the overall health and well-being of the host. The gut microbiome is often referred to as a "forgotten organ" because of its significant impact on various physiological processes.

The human gut is home to trillions of microorganisms, with bacterial cells outnumbering human cells by approximately 10 to 1. These microorganisms harbor a complex and dynamic ecosystem that begins to establish itself at birth and continues to evolve throughout a person's life. The composition of the gut microbiome is influenced by factors such as genetics, diet, environment, and lifestyle. A balanced and diverse gut microbiome is crucial for maintaining health, whereas imbalances in this microbial community can lead to various health issues.

Functions of Gut Bacteria

Gut bacteria play numerous vital roles in the body, impacting everything from digestion to immune function and mental health. Some of the key functions of gut bacteria include:

1. Digestion and Nutrient Absorption

Gut bacteria help break down complex carbohydrates, proteins, and fats that the human digestive enzymes cannot completely process. They ferment dietary fibers into short-chain fatty acids (SCFAs) like butyrate, acetate, and propionate, which are essential for maintaining gut health and providing energy to colon cells.

2. Synthesis of Vitamins

Certain gut bacteria are involved in the synthesis of essential vitamins, including vitamin K and some B vitamins (B12, riboflavin, and folate). These vitamins are critical for blood coagulation, energy metabolism, and various cellular functions.

3. Immune System Modulation

The gut microbiome plays a crucial role in training and modulating the immune system. It helps distinguish between harmful pathogens and benign or beneficial microorganisms, reducing the risk of autoimmune diseases and allergies. Gut bacteria also produce antimicrobial peptides that protect against pathogenic microbes.

4. Protection Against Pathogens

Beneficial gut bacteria inhibit the growth of pathogenic bacteria by competing for nutrients and attachment sites on the gut lining. They also produce substances like bacteriocins and SCFAs that directly inhibit pathogen growth.

5. Regulation of Metabolism

Gut bacteria influence host metabolism by affecting the storage and utilization of fats. They play a role in energy balance and may impact conditions such as obesity, diabetes, and metabolic syndrome.

6. Mental Health and Mood Regulation

The gut-brain axis is a bidirectional communication system between the gut and the brain, mediated by the nervous system, hormones, and immune molecules. Gut bacteria produce neurotransmitters like serotonin and gamma-aminobutyric acid (GABA), which can influence mood, anxiety, and cognitive function.

The Role of Probiotics and Prebiotics

Probiotics

Probiotics are live microorganisms that confer health benefits to the host when consumed in adequate amounts. They are found in various fermented foods and dietary supplements. Common probiotic strains include Lactobacillus, Bifidobacterium, and Saccharomyces. Probiotics help restore and maintain a healthy gut microbiome, especially after disruptions caused by illness or antibiotic use.

Benefits of Probiotics

- Restoring Gut Balance: Probiotics can help replenish beneficial bacteria, restoring balance to the gut microbiome after disruptions.
- Enhancing Immune Function: Probiotics modulate

the immune system, enhancing its ability to fight off infections and reducing inflammation.

- Improving Digestive Health: Probiotics can alleviate symptoms of gastrointestinal disorders such as irritable bowel syndrome (IBS), diarrhea, and constipation.
- Supporting Mental Health: Some probiotic strains have been shown to reduce symptoms of anxiety and depression through their impact on the gut-brain axis.

Prebiotics

Prebiotics are non-digestible food components that selectively stimulate the growth and activity of beneficial gut bacteria. They are typically found in high-fiber foods such as garlic, onions, leeks, asparagus, bananas, and whole grains. Prebiotics serve as a food source for probiotics, promoting their growth and activity in the gut.

Benefits of Prebiotics

- Promoting Beneficial Bacteria: Prebiotics enhance the growth and activity of probiotics, supporting a healthy gut microbiome.
- Improving Digestive Health: By increasing the production of SCFAs, prebiotics help maintain gut barrier integrity and reduce inflammation.
- Supporting Immune Function: Prebiotics modulate the immune system, improving its response to infections and reducing the risk of chronic diseases.

- Enhancing Mineral Absorption: Prebiotics can improve the absorption of minerals such as calcium and magnesium, supporting bone health.

Impact of Antibiotics on Gut Health

While antibiotics are essential for treating bacterial infections, their use can have a significant impact on the gut microbiome. Antibiotics do not discriminate between harmful pathogens and beneficial bacteria, leading to a reduction in microbial diversity and the disruption of the gut ecosystem. This disruption, known as dysbiosis, can result in several negative consequences:

Short-Term Effects

Digestive Issues: Antibiotic use can lead to diarrhea, nausea, and abdominal pain as the balance of gut bacteria is disrupted.
Opportunistic Infections: A reduction in beneficial bacteria can create an opportunity for harmful bacteria like Clostridium difficile (C. difficile) to proliferate, causing severe infections.

Long-Term Effects

Reduced Microbial Diversity: Repeated or prolonged antibiotic use can lead to a long-term decrease in microbial diversity, which is associated with various health issues.
Increased Risk of Chronic Diseases: Dysbiosis

resulting from antibiotic use has been linked to an increased risk of conditions such as obesity, diabetes, inflammatory bowel disease, and allergies.
Antibiotic Resistance: Overuse of antibiotics can contribute to the development of antibiotic-resistant bacteria, making infections harder to treat.

Mitigating the Impact

To mitigate the impact of antibiotics on gut health, it is important to use antibiotics judiciously and only when necessary. Additionally, incorporating probiotics and prebiotics into the diet can help restore and maintain a healthy gut microbiome during and after antibiotic treatment.

How Lifestyle Affects the Microbiome

The health and composition of the gut microbiome are influenced by various lifestyle factors beyond diet. These include physical activity, sleep, stress management, and exposure to environmental toxins.

Physical Activity

Regular physical activity has been shown to positively influence gut health. Exercise increases microbial diversity and promotes the growth of beneficial bacteria. It also enhances gut motility and reduces the risk of gastrointestinal disorders.

Sleep

Quality sleep is essential for maintaining a healthy gut microbiome. Disruptions in sleep patterns can lead to changes in gut bacteria composition, contributing to dysbiosis and inflammation. Establishing a regular sleep routine and ensuring adequate rest can support gut health.

Stress Management

Chronic stress negatively impacts gut health by altering the gut microbiome and increasing intestinal permeability. Stress management techniques such as mindfulness, meditation, and regular physical activity can help mitigate these effects and promote a healthy gut.

Environmental Toxins

Exposure to environmental toxins, such as pesticides, heavy metals, and pollutants, can disrupt the gut microbiome and contribute to dysbiosis. Reducing exposure to these toxins through dietary choices, water filtration, and minimizing the use of chemical-based products can support gut health.

Importance of Diversity in Gut Bacteria

Diversity in the gut microbiome is a key indicator of health. A diverse microbial community is more resilient and better able to perform essential functions, including digestion, immune modulation, and protection against pathogens. Conversely, a lack of diversity is associated with various health issues and increased susceptibility to diseases.

Benefits of Microbial Diversity

- Enhanced Resilience: A diverse microbiome is more adaptable and better able to withstand disruptions such as illness, antibiotic use, and dietary changes.
- Improved Digestion and Nutrient Absorption: A wider variety of bacteria enhances the ability to break down and assimilate different nutrients, supporting overall health.
- Balanced Immune Function: Microbial diversity helps regulate immune responses, reducing the risk of autoimmune and inflammatory diseases.
- Protection Against Pathogens: A diverse microbiome is more effective at inhibiting the growth of harmful bacteria and preventing infections.

Strategies to Promote Microbial Diversity

- Varied Diet: Consuming a wide range of plant-based foods, rich in fiber and prebiotics, supports microbial diversity.
- Fermented Foods: Including a variety of fermented foods in the diet introduces beneficial bacteria and promotes microbial diversity.
- Limiting Antibiotic Use: Using antibiotics only

when necessary and under medical supervision helps preserve microbial diversity.

- Stress Management: Reducing stress through mindfulness, relaxation techniques, and physical activity supports a healthy and diverse microbiome.
- Exposure to Nature: Spending time in natural environments and interacting with pets can increase exposure to diverse microorganisms, promoting gut health.

In conclusion, understanding the gut microbiome and its profound impact on health is essential for making informed dietary and lifestyle choices. By prioritizing gut health through balanced nutrition, mindful lifestyle practices, and targeted interventions, individuals can support a thriving gut microbiome and enhance their overall well-being.

Chapter 02

Identifying and Avoiding Gut Disruptors

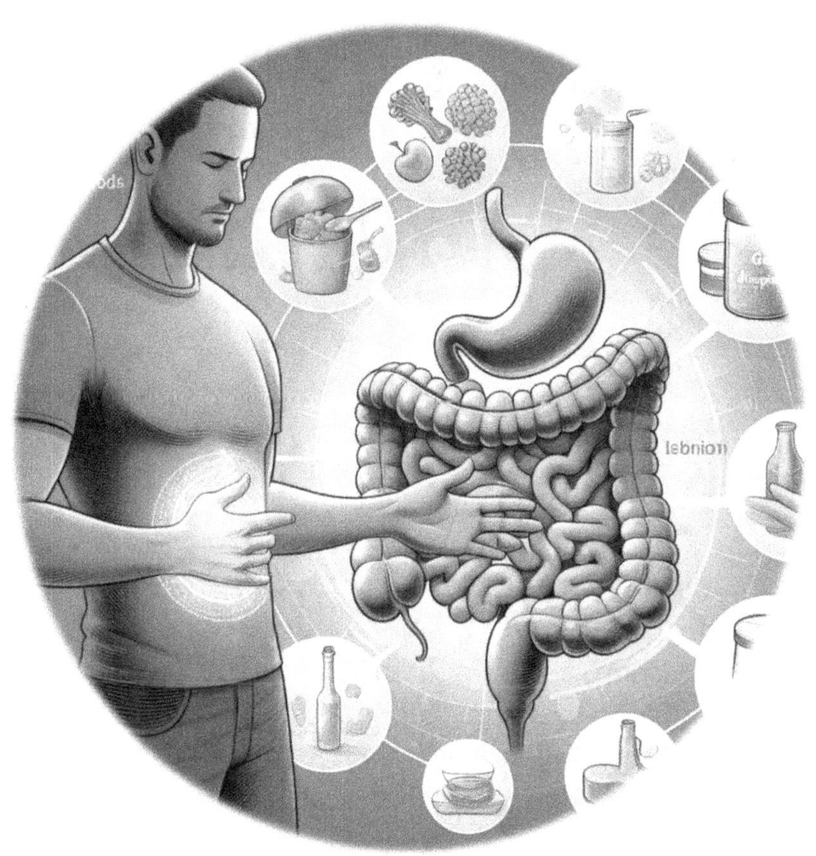

Common Dietary Gut Disruptors

The modern diet is rife with dietary gut disruptors that can wreak havoc on the delicate balance of the gut microbiome and compromise digestive health. Understanding these common culprits is essential for making informed dietary choices and safeguarding gut health.

Sugar

Excessive consumption of refined sugars and high-fructose corn syrup is a major contributor to gut disruption. These sugars provide fuel for pathogenic bacteria and yeast in the gut, leading to dysbiosis and inflammation. Moreover, a high sugar intake can impair gut barrier function and increase intestinal permeability, commonly referred to as "leaky gut syndrome."

Processed Foods

Processed foods, characterized by their high levels of refined grains, added sugars, unhealthy fats, and artificial additives, are detrimental to gut health. These foods lack the essential nutrients and fiber needed to support a healthy microbiome, while their additives can disrupt microbial balance and promote inflammation.

Artificial Sweeteners

Artificial sweeteners, commonly found in diet sodas, sugar-free snacks, and processed foods, have been linked to gut dysbiosis and metabolic disturbances. Despite their zero-calorie appeal, artificial sweeteners can alter gut bacteria composition, increase glucose intolerance, and promote weight gain.

Industrial Seed Oils

Industrial seed oils like soybean oil, corn oil, and canola oil are rich in omega-6 fatty acids and prone to oxidation, contributing to inflammation and oxidative stress in the gut. These oils are commonly used in processed and fried foods, making them prevalent in the Western diet.

Food Additives and Preservatives

Artificial food additives and preservatives, such as emulsifiers, stabilizers, and synthetic colors, can disrupt gut microbiota composition and integrity. These chemicals have been shown to increase intestinal permeability and promote inflammation, contributing to gut dysfunction and associated health issues.

Environmental Factors Affecting Gut Health

Beyond dietary choices, various environmental factors can impact gut health and contribute to gut disruption. Understanding and minimizing exposure to these factors is crucial for supporting optimal digestive function and overall well-being.

Environmental Toxins

Exposure to environmental toxins, including pesticides, heavy metals, air pollutants, and industrial chemicals, can disrupt the gut microbiome and impair gastrointestinal health. Minimizing exposure through organic food choices, water filtration, and toxin-free household products can mitigate these risks.

Pollution and Urbanization

Urbanization and pollution can negatively impact gut health by altering microbial diversity and promoting inflammation. Studies have shown that urban dwellers have less diverse gut microbiota compared to rural populations, likely due to differences in diet, lifestyle, and environmental exposures.

Antibiotic Resistance

The widespread use of antibiotics in agriculture, veterinary medicine, and human healthcare has led to the emergence of antibiotic-resistant bacteria, posing a significant threat to gut health and microbial balance. Resistant bacteria can proliferate in the gut, displacing beneficial microbes and increasing the risk of infections and antibiotic-associated complications.

The Role of Stress and Sleep

Stress and sleep play integral roles in gut health, with chronic stress and sleep disturbances contributing to gut disruption and digestive disorders.

Stress

Chronic stress can disrupt gut microbiota composition, impair gut barrier function, and promote inflammation, leading to gastrointestinal symptoms such as bloating, diarrhea, and abdominal pain. Stress management techniques such as mindfulness, meditation, and deep breathing exercises can help mitigate these effects and support gut health.

Sleep

Quality sleep is essential for gut health, with inadequate sleep linked to alterations in gut microbiota composition, increased intestinal permeability, and heightened inflammation. Establishing a regular sleep schedule, practicing good sleep hygiene, and prioritizing relaxation can promote optimal gut function and overall well-being.

Medications and Their Impact on the Gut

Certain medications can disrupt gut health by altering microbial balance, impairing gut barrier function, and promoting inflammation. Understanding the potential effects of these medications is essential for minimizing their impact on digestive health.

Antibiotics

While antibiotics are crucial for treating bacterial infections, their use can lead to gut dysbiosis and associated digestive issues. Antibiotics indiscriminately target both harmful and beneficial bacteria, disrupting microbial balance and increasing the risk of antibiotic-associated complications such as diarrhea and Clostridium difficile infection.

Non-Steroidal Anti-Inflammatory Drugs (NSAIDs)

Non-steroidal anti-inflammatory drugs (NSAIDs) like ibuprofen and aspirin can irritate the gastrointestinal lining, leading to mucosal damage, increased intestinal permeability, and gut inflammation. Prolonged NSAID use is associated with an increased risk of gastrointestinal complications such as ulcers, bleeding, and inflammatory bowel disease.

Proton Pump Inhibitors (PPIs)

Proton pump inhibitors (PPIs) are commonly prescribed to reduce gastric acid production and treat conditions such as acid reflux and peptic ulcers. However, long-term PPI use can alter gut microbiota composition, increase the risk of small intestinal bacterial overgrowth (SIBO), and impair nutrient absorption.

Symptoms of Gut Disruption

Identifying the signs of gut disruption is essential for recognizing potential digestive issues and taking proactive steps to restore gut health. Common symptoms of gut disruption include:

- Digestive Issues: Chronic bloating, gas, diarrhea, constipation, and abdominal discomfort.
- Food Intolerances: Difficulty digesting certain foods, leading to symptoms like bloating, cramps, and diarrhea.
- Immune Dysfunction: Frequent infections, allergies, and autoimmune reactions.
- Skin Conditions: Eczema, acne, and psoriasis may indicate underlying gut issues and inflammation.
- Mood Disorders: Anxiety, depression, irritability, and mood swings may be linked to gut-brain axis dysfunction.
- Fatigue and Low Energy: Chronic fatigue, lethargy,

and low energy levels can result from poor nutrient absorption and inflammation.

Steps to Eliminate or Reduce Disruptors

To promote gut health and minimize gut disruptors, consider implementing the following strategies:

- Adopt a Whole Foods Diet: Focus on whole, unprocessed foods rich in fiber, vitamins, and minerals to support gut health and microbial balance.
- Reduce Sugar and Processed Foods: Limit intake of refined sugars, processed foods, and artificial additives that can disrupt gut microbiota composition and promote inflammation.
- Manage Stress: Practice stress-reduction techniques such as mindfulness, meditation, yoga, and deep breathing exercises to support gut health and overall well-being.
- Prioritize Sleep: Aim for 7-9 hours of quality sleep per night to promote optimal gut function, repair, and regeneration.
- Use Medications Judiciously: Use antibiotics, NSAIDs, and other medications only when necessary and under medical supervision to minimize their impact on gut health.
- Seek Professional Guidance: Consult with a healthcare provider or registered dietitian for personalized recommendations and guidance on

supporting gut health through diet, lifestyle, and targeted interventions.

By identifying and avoiding common gut disruptors, individuals can take proactive steps to support digestive health, optimize gut function, and enhance overall well-being. Prioritizing gut health through mindful dietary choices, stress management, and healthy lifestyle habits lays the foundation for vibrant health and vitality.

Chapter 03

Boosting Fiber Intake

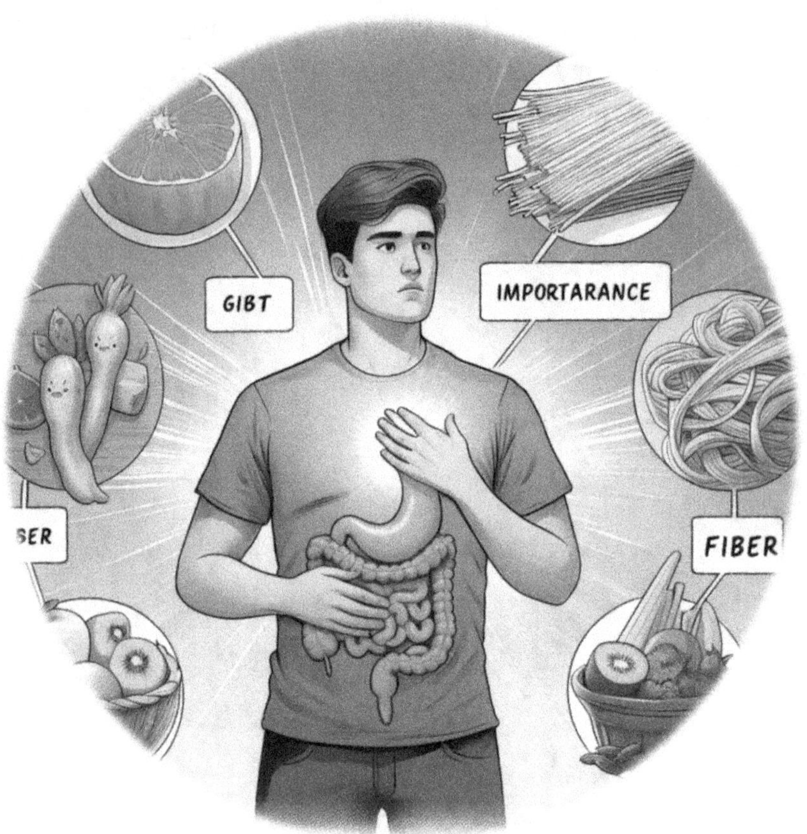

Fiber serves as an unsung hero in the realm of nutrition, often overlooked but essential for maintaining optimal gut health and overall well-being. In this chapter, we will delve deeper into the importance of fiber, explore the different types of fiber, highlight the best food sources of fiber, discuss daily intake recommendations, and provide practical tips for increasing fiber in your diet. Additionally, we will explore the use of fiber supplements, including when and how to incorporate them into your wellness routine.

Importance of Fiber for Gut Health

Fiber, a type of carbohydrate found in plant-based foods, plays a crucial role in supporting digestive health and promoting overall wellness. Unlike other nutrients, fiber is not digested by the body but instead passes through the digestive tract relatively intact, exerting numerous beneficial effects along the way.

Key Benefits of Fiber for Gut Health:

- Promotes Regular Bowel Movements: Fiber adds bulk to stools, softening them and facilitating bowel movements. This helps prevent constipation and promotes digestive regularity, supporting overall gut health.

- Supports Gut Microbiome: Certain types of fiber, known as prebiotics, serve as food for beneficial gut bacteria. By nourishing these microbes, fiber helps maintain a healthy balance of gut flora, which is essential for digestion, immune function, and overall well-being.

- Aids in Weight Management: Fiber-rich foods tend to be more filling and satisfying, which can help control appetite and reduce overall calorie intake. By promoting feelings of fullness, fiber supports weight management and may aid in weight loss efforts.

- Regulates Blood Sugar Levels: Soluble fiber, in particular, can help stabilize blood sugar levels by slowing the absorption of glucose from the digestive tract. This can help prevent spikes and crashes in blood sugar, promoting stable energy levels and reducing the risk of type 2 diabetes.

- Supports Heart Health: High-fiber diets have been associated with a reduced risk of heart disease and stroke. Fiber helps lower cholesterol levels, reduce blood pressure, and improve markers of cardiovascular health, making it an essential component of a heart-healthy diet.

Types of Fiber: Soluble and Insoluble

Fiber can be classified into two main types based on its solubility in water: soluble fiber and insoluble fiber. Each type of fiber has unique properties and health benefits, and both are important for supporting digestive health and overall wellness.

Soluble Fiber:

Soluble fiber dissolves in water to form a gel-like substance in the digestive tract. This type of fiber is fermented by beneficial gut bacteria in the colon, producing short-chain fatty acids (SCFAs) that nourish colon cells and support gut health. Good sources of soluble fiber include oats, barley, legumes, apples, citrus fruits, and flaxseeds.

Soluble fiber has been shown to:

- Lower cholesterol levels by binding to bile acids and promoting their excretion from the body.
- Stabilize blood sugar levels by slowing the absorption of glucose from the digestive tract.
- Promote feelings of fullness and satiety, which can aid in weight management and appetite control.

Insoluble Fiber:

Insoluble fiber does not dissolve in water and passes through the digestive tract largely intact. It adds bulk to stools and helps promote regular bowel movements by speeding up the passage of food through the intestines. Foods rich in insoluble fiber include whole grains, nuts, seeds, vegetables, and fruit skins.

Insoluble fiber has been shown to:

- Promote regular bowel movements and prevent

constipation by adding bulk to stools and speeding up intestinal transit time.
- Help maintain bowel health by reducing the risk of diverticulosis and hemorrhoids.
- Support overall digestive health by providing roughage and stimulating peristalsis, the wave-like contractions of the intestines that propel food through the digestive tract.

Best Food Sources of Fiber

A wide variety of whole foods are rich sources of fiber, providing both soluble and insoluble forms of this essential nutrient. Incorporating a diverse range of fiber-rich foods into your diet can help ensure an adequate intake of fiber and support optimal digestive health.

High-Fiber Foods:

- Whole Grains: Whole grains such as quinoa, brown rice, barley, bulgur, and whole wheat pasta are excellent sources of fiber. Opt for whole grains over refined grains to maximize fiber intake and nutritional benefits.

- Legumes: Beans, lentils, chickpeas, and split peas are rich sources of both soluble and insoluble fiber. Incorporate legumes into soups, stews, salads, and casseroles for a hearty dose of fiber and plant-based protein.

- Fruits: Berries, apples, pears, oranges, bananas, and avocados are all excellent sources of fiber. Enjoy fruits fresh, frozen, or dried as a nutritious snack or incorporate them into smoothies, yogurt, oatmeal, or salads for added fiber and flavor.

- Vegetables: Broccoli, Brussels sprouts, spinach, kale, carrots, sweet potatoes, and cauliflower are all rich sources of fiber. Include a variety of colorful vegetables in your meals to maximize fiber intake and nutritional diversity.

- Nuts and Seeds: Almonds, chia seeds, flaxseeds, pumpkin seeds, and sunflower seeds are packed with fiber, healthy fats, and essential nutrients. Enjoy nuts and seeds as a snack or sprinkle them on salads, yogurt, oatmeal, or baked goods for added crunch and fiber.

Daily Fiber Intake Recommendations

The recommended daily intake of fiber varies based on age, sex, and individual dietary needs. However, most health organizations provide general guidelines for fiber intake to support optimal health and digestive function.

Dietary Guidelines for Americans (2020-2025):

- Adult Men (ages 19-50): 38 grams of fiber per day.
- Adult Women (ages 19-50): 25 grams of fiber per day.

- Adults Over 50: Men should aim for 30 grams of fiber per day, while women should aim for 21 grams.
- Meeting these recommendations can help support digestive regularity, maintain a healthy gut microbiome, and reduce the risk of chronic diseases such as heart disease, diabetes, and certain types of cancer.

Easy Ways to Increase Fiber in Your Diet

Incorporating more fiber into your diet doesn't have to be complicated. With a few simple strategies, you can boost your fiber intake and enjoy the health benefits of this essential nutrient.

Tips for Increasing Fiber Intake:

1. Choose Whole Foods: Opt for whole, minimally processed foods whenever possible. Whole grains, fruits, vegetables, legumes, nuts, and seeds are all excellent sources of fiber and other essential nutrients.

2. Eat Plenty of Fruits and Vegetables: Aim to fill half your plate with fruits and vegetables at each meal. Choose a variety of colors and types to maximize fiber intake and nutritional diversity.

3. Include Fiber-Rich Snacks: Snack on fiber-rich foods like fresh fruit, raw vegetables, nuts, and

seeds throughout the day to boost fiber intake and satisfy hunger between meals.

4. Swap Refined Grains for Whole Grains: Replace refined grains like white bread, white rice, and regular pasta with whole grains such as whole wheat bread, brown rice, quinoa, and whole wheat pasta. Whole grains are higher in fiber and provide additional nutrients such as vitamins, minerals, and antioxidants.

5. Add Beans and Legumes to Meals: Incorporate beans, lentils, chickpeas, and other legumes into soups, stews, salads, and casseroles. These versatile plant-based proteins are rich in fiber and can help boost satiety and promote digestive health.

6. Snack on Nuts and Seeds: Enjoy a handful of nuts or seeds as a nutritious snack or add them to yogurt, oatmeal, or salads for extra crunch and fiber. Almonds, chia seeds, flaxseeds, and pumpkin seeds are all excellent choices.

7. Start Your Day with Fiber: Kickstart your morning with a fiber-rich breakfast. Oatmeal topped with fresh fruit, whole grain toast with avocado, or a smoothie made with leafy greens and berries are all delicious and nutritious options.

8. Incorporate Fiber-Rich Foods into Recipes: Get creative in the kitchen and incorporate fiber-rich

ingredients into your favorite recipes. Add vegetables to omelets, soups, and stir-fries, swap refined grains for whole grains in baking recipes, and experiment with legumes in tacos, chili, and pasta dishes.

By making small changes to your diet and incorporating more fiber-rich foods into your meals and snacks, you can easily increase your fiber intake and reap the health benefits of this essential nutrient.

Fiber Supplements: When and How to Use Them

While whole foods are the best sources of fiber, fiber supplements can be a convenient option for individuals who struggle to meet their fiber needs through diet alone or have specific digestive issues that may benefit from additional fiber. Fiber supplements come in various forms, including powders, capsules, chewable tablets, and gummies, and may contain soluble fiber, insoluble fiber, or a combination of both.

When to Consider Fiber Supplements:

1. Insufficient Fiber Intake: If you consistently fall short of meeting your daily fiber needs through diet alone, a fiber supplement can help bridge the gap and ensure you're getting enough fiber to support optimal digestive health.

2. Constipation: Fiber supplements can be particularly beneficial for individuals who struggle with constipation or irregular bowel movements. Soluble fiber supplements, in particular, can help soften stools and promote regularity.

3. Digestive Disorders: Certain digestive disorders, such as irritable bowel syndrome (IBS), inflammatory bowel disease (IBD), and diverticulosis, may benefit from fiber supplementation. However, it's essential to consult with a healthcare provider before starting a fiber supplement, as individual needs and tolerances may vary.

How to Use Fiber Supplements:

1. Start Slowly: If you're new to fiber supplements, start with a low dose and gradually increase the dose over time. This allows your digestive system to adjust gradually and helps minimize the risk of gastrointestinal discomfort such as bloating, gas, and cramping.

2. Stay Hydrated: Fiber supplements absorb water in the digestive tract, so it's essential to drink plenty of fluids when taking them. Aim to drink at least eight glasses of water per day to help prevent dehydration and support optimal digestion.

3. Follow Dosage Recommendations: Follow the manufacturer's dosage recommendations and any

guidance provided by your healthcare provider or registered dietitian. It's essential to take fiber supplements as directed to ensure safety and effectiveness.

4. Monitor Symptoms: Pay attention to how your body responds to the fiber supplement. If you experience any adverse reactions or digestive discomfort, discontinue use and consult with a healthcare professional.

5. Consider Timing: Some people find it helpful to take fiber supplements with meals or snacks to minimize the risk of gastrointestinal discomfort. Experiment with different timing options to find what works best for you.

In conclusion, fiber is a vital nutrient for supporting digestive health, promoting regularity, and reducing the risk of chronic diseases. By incorporating more fiber-rich foods into your diet and considering fiber supplements when needed, you can boost your fiber intake and enjoy the many health benefits this essential nutrient has to offer. Remember to start slowly with fiber supplements, stay hydrated, and listen to your body's cues to ensure a positive and comfortable experience. If you have any questions or concerns about fiber supplementation, be sure to consult with a healthcare provider or registered dietitian for personalized guidance and recommendations.

Chapter 04

The Anti-Inflammatory Diet

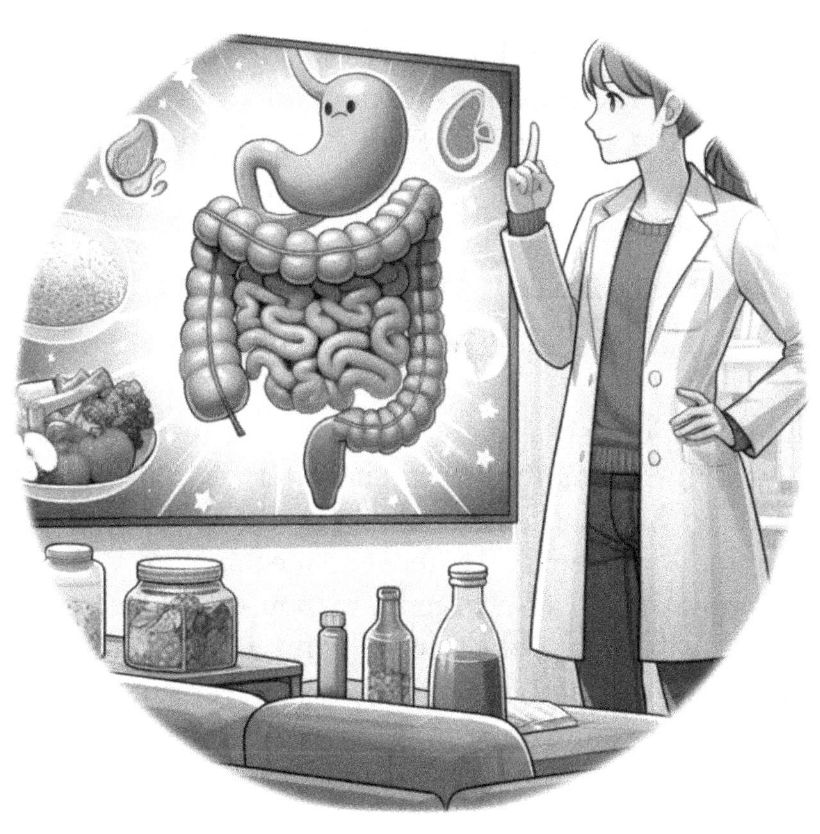

Inflammation is a natural and essential response of the immune system to injury, infection, or tissue damage. However, chronic inflammation, often driven by factors such as poor diet, stress, and lifestyle habits, can contribute to a host of health issues, including digestive disorders, autoimmune conditions, and cardiovascular disease. In this chapter, we will explore the concept of inflammation and its impact on gut health, discuss the principles of an anti-inflammatory diet, highlight foods to include and avoid, provide guidance on balancing omega-3 and omega-6 fatty acids, offer a sample anti-inflammatory meal plan, and examine the long-term benefits of adopting an anti-inflammatory diet.

Understanding Inflammation and Its Impact on the Gut

Inflammation is the body's natural response to injury, infection, or irritation. It is characterized by redness, swelling, heat, and pain and is a crucial part of the immune system's defense mechanism. Acute inflammation is a short-term response that helps the body heal and protect itself from harm. However, chronic inflammation, which persists over time, can be harmful and contribute to a range of health problems, including gastrointestinal issues.

Chronic inflammation in the gut can disrupt the delicate balance of the gut microbiome, impair gut barrier function, and contribute to conditions such as irritable bowel syndrome (IBS), inflammatory bowel disease (IBD), and leaky gut syndrome. By adopting an anti-inflammatory diet and lifestyle, you can help reduce inflammation in the gut and support digestive health.

Anti-Inflammatory Foods and Their Benefits

An anti-inflammatory diet focuses on consuming whole, nutrient-dense foods that have been shown to reduce inflammation in the body. These foods are rich in antioxidants, vitamins, minerals, and phytonutrients that help combat oxidative stress and inflammation. Incorporating a variety of anti-inflammatory foods into your diet can help support gut health, reduce inflammation, and promote overall well-being.

Key Anti-Inflammatory Foods:

- Fatty Fish: Fatty fish such as salmon, mackerel, sardines, and trout are rich in omega-3 fatty acids, which have potent anti-inflammatory properties. Consuming fatty fish regularly can help reduce inflammation in the body and support heart health.

- Berries: Berries such as blueberries, strawberries, raspberries, and blackberries are packed with antioxidants, including flavonoids and anthocyanins, which help combat inflammation and oxidative stress.

- Leafy Greens: Leafy greens such as spinach, kale, Swiss chard, and collard greens are excellent sources of vitamins, minerals, and phytonutrients that help reduce inflammation and support overall health.

- Turmeric: Turmeric contains a compound called curcumin, which has powerful anti-inflammatory and antioxidant properties. Adding turmeric to your meals or enjoying turmeric tea can help reduce inflammation and promote healing in the body.

- Olive Oil: Extra virgin olive oil is rich in monounsaturated fats and contains antioxidants such as oleocanthal, which help reduce inflammation and support heart health. Use olive oil as your primary cooking oil or drizzle it over salads and vegetables for added flavor and health benefits.

- Nuts and Seeds: Nuts and seeds such as almonds, walnuts, flaxseeds, and chia seeds are rich in healthy fats, fiber, and antioxidants, which help reduce inflammation and support gut health.

- Colorful Vegetables: Colorful vegetables such as bell peppers, tomatoes, carrots, and sweet potatoes are rich in vitamins, minerals, and antioxidants that help reduce inflammation and support overall health.

- Green Tea: Green tea contains catechins, which are powerful antioxidants that help reduce inflammation and support immune function. Enjoying a cup of green tea regularly can help promote gut health and reduce inflammation in the body.

Foods to Avoid to Reduce Inflammation

In addition to incorporating anti-inflammatory foods into your diet, it's essential to limit or avoid foods that can promote inflammation and contribute to gut health issues. These include processed foods, refined carbohydrates, sugary snacks and beverages, fried foods, and foods high in trans fats and artificial additives.

Key Inflammatory Foods to Avoid:

- Refined Sugars: Refined sugars found in processed foods, sugary snacks, and sweetened beverages can promote inflammation and contribute to gut health issues. Limiting your intake of refined sugars and opting for natural sweeteners such as honey or maple syrup can help reduce inflammation in the body.

- Processed Foods: Processed foods such as fast food, frozen meals, and packaged snacks are often high in unhealthy fats, refined carbohydrates, and artificial additives, all of which can promote inflammation and contribute to gut health issues. Choosing whole, minimally processed foods whenever possible is key to reducing inflammation and supporting digestive health.

- Trans Fats: Trans fats, found in partially hydrogenated oils used in fried foods, baked goods, and processed snacks, are highly inflammatory and can contribute to heart disease, diabetes, and other health problems. Avoiding foods high in trans fats and opting for healthier fats such as olive oil, avocado, and nuts can help reduce inflammation and support overall health.

- Highly Processed Oils: Highly processed oils such as corn oil, soybean oil, and vegetable oil are high in omega-6 fatty acids, which can promote inflammation when consumed in excess. Limiting your intake of these oils and choosing healthier fats such as olive oil, avocado oil, and coconut oil can help reduce inflammation in the body.

- Artificial Additives: Artificial additives such as artificial colors, flavors, and preservatives found in processed foods and beverages can promote inflammation and contribute to gut health issues. Choosing whole, natural foods and reading labels carefully can help minimize your exposure to these additives and reduce inflammation in the body.

- How to Balance Omega-3 and Omega-6 Fatty Acids

- Balancing omega-3 and omega-6 fatty acids is essential for reducing inflammation and supporting overall health. While both omega-3 and omega-6 fatty acids are necessary for optimal health, the typical Western diet tends to be high in omega-6 fatty acids and low in omega-3 fatty acids, which can promote inflammation and contribute to chronic disease.

Tips for Balancing Omega-3 and Omega-6 Fatty Acids:

1. Increase Omega-3-Rich Foods: Incorporate more omega-3-rich foods into your diet, such as fatty fish (salmon, mackerel, sardines), flaxseeds, chia seeds, hemp seeds, walnuts, and algae-based supplements. These foods contain alpha-linolenic acid (ALA), a type of omega-3 fatty acid that helps reduce inflammation and support heart health.

2. Reduce Omega-6-Rich Foods: Limit your intake of omega-6-rich foods, such as processed oils (corn oil, soybean oil, vegetable oil), fried foods, processed snacks, and conventionally raised meats. These foods are high in linoleic acid, a type of omega-6 fatty acid that can promote inflammation when consumed in excess.

3. Choose Healthy Cooking Oils: Opt for healthier cooking oils such as olive oil, avocado oil, and coconut oil, which are lower in omega-6 fatty acids and higher in monounsaturated fats or saturated

fats. These oils are less likely to promote inflammation and can help balance omega-3 and omega-6 fatty acids in the diet.

4. Read Food Labels: Be mindful of food labels and ingredient lists when shopping for packaged foods. Avoid products that contain hydrogenated or partially hydrogenated oils, which are sources of unhealthy trans fats. Instead, choose products made with healthier fats and oils.

5. Cook at Home: Cooking meals at home allows you to have more control over the ingredients you use and the cooking methods employed. Opt for cooking techniques such as baking, grilling, steaming, or sautéing with healthier oils to minimize the intake of inflammatory fats.

6. Supplement Wisely: Consider incorporating omega-3 supplements into your routine if you struggle to obtain sufficient amounts through dietary sources alone. Fish oil supplements, algae oil supplements (for vegetarians and vegans), or krill oil supplements can provide concentrated doses of EPA (eicosapentaenoic acid) and DHA (docosahexaenoic acid), two types of omega-3 fatty acids with potent anti-inflammatory properties.

Sample Anti-Inflammatory Meal Plan

Creating a meal plan that incorporates anti-inflammatory foods can help simplify your journey toward better gut health and reduced inflammation. Below is a sample one-day meal plan that highlights nourishing, anti-inflammatory foods and demonstrates how to incorporate them into your daily routine.

Breakfast:

- Turmeric Oatmeal: Start your day with a warming bowl of turmeric oatmeal. Cook rolled oats with almond milk, a pinch of turmeric, cinnamon, and ginger until creamy. Top with fresh berries, sliced bananas, chopped walnuts, and a drizzle of honey for added sweetness and anti-inflammatory benefits.

Mid-Morning Snack:

- Greek Yogurt Parfait: Enjoy a Greek yogurt parfait layered with fresh berries, almonds, and a sprinkle of ground flaxseeds. Greek yogurt is rich in probiotics, which support gut health, while berries provide antioxidants and fiber to combat inflammation.

Lunch:

- Salmon Salad: Prepare a salmon salad with mixed greens, grilled or baked salmon fillet, cherry tomatoes, cucumber slices, avocado, and pumpkin seeds. Dress with a simple vinaigrette made from extra virgin olive oil, lemon juice, Dijon mustard, and a pinch of sea salt. The salmon provides omega-3 fatty acids to reduce inflammation, while the vegetables offer a variety of vitamins, minerals, and antioxidants.

Afternoon Snack:

- Carrot Sticks with Hummus: Enjoy a crunchy and satisfying snack of carrot sticks dipped in hummus. Carrots are rich in beta-carotene, a powerful antioxidant, while hummus provides fiber, protein, and healthy fats to keep you feeling full and satisfied until dinner.

Dinner:

- Quinoa Stir-Fry: Whip up a quick and nutritious quinoa stir-fry with mixed vegetables, tofu or chicken breast, and a homemade stir-fry sauce. Use a combination of colorful vegetables such as bell peppers, broccoli, snap peas, and carrots for maximum nutritional benefits. Quinoa serves as a gluten-free source of protein and fiber, while the vegetables and lean protein provide essential nutrients and anti-inflammatory compounds.

Evening Snack:

- Mixed Nuts: Enjoy a handful of mixed nuts such as almonds, walnuts, and cashews as a satisfying evening snack. Nuts are rich in healthy fats, protein, and fiber, which help stabilize blood sugar levels and reduce inflammation in the body.

Long-Term Benefits of an Anti-Inflammatory Diet

Adopting an anti-inflammatory diet can offer numerous long-term benefits for gut health, overall well-being, and disease prevention. By focusing on whole, nutrient-dense foods and minimizing inflammatory foods and beverages, you can:

- Reduce Chronic Inflammation: An anti-inflammatory diet helps reduce chronic inflammation in the body, which can alleviate symptoms of inflammatory conditions such as arthritis, IBS, and autoimmune diseases.

- Support Digestive Health: By promoting a healthy balance of gut microbiota, strengthening gut barrier function, and reducing inflammation in the gut, an anti-inflammatory diet supports optimal digestive health and reduces the risk of digestive disorders.

- Promote Heart Health: Consuming anti-inflammatory foods such as fatty fish, olive oil, nuts, and berries can help lower cholesterol levels, reduce blood pressure, and decrease the risk of heart disease and stroke.

- Maintain a Healthy Weight: An anti-inflammatory diet rich in fiber, lean protein, and healthy fats can help regulate appetite, promote feelings of fullness, and support weight management and maintenance.

- Boost Immune Function: Many anti-inflammatory foods are rich in vitamins, minerals, and antioxidants that support immune function and help protect against infections and illness.

- Enhance Overall Well-Being: By nourishing your body with nutrient-dense foods and minimizing exposure to inflammatory substances, an anti-inflammatory diet can enhance overall well-being, increase energy levels, and improve mood and mental clarity.

In conclusion, an anti-inflammatory diet is a powerful tool for promoting gut health, reducing inflammation, and supporting overall well-being. By focusing on whole, nutrient-dense foods such as fatty fish, berries, leafy greens, and nuts, and minimizing inflammatory foods such as processed snacks, refined sugars, and trans fats, you can optimize your diet for gut health and long-term wellness. Remember to listen to your body, experiment with different foods and recipes, and seek guidance from a healthcare professional or registered dietitian if you have specific dietary concerns or health conditions. With mindful food choices and a commitment to nourishing your body with anti-inflammatory foods, you can take proactive steps toward better gut health and a vibrant, thriving life.

Chapter 05

Hydration and Gut Health

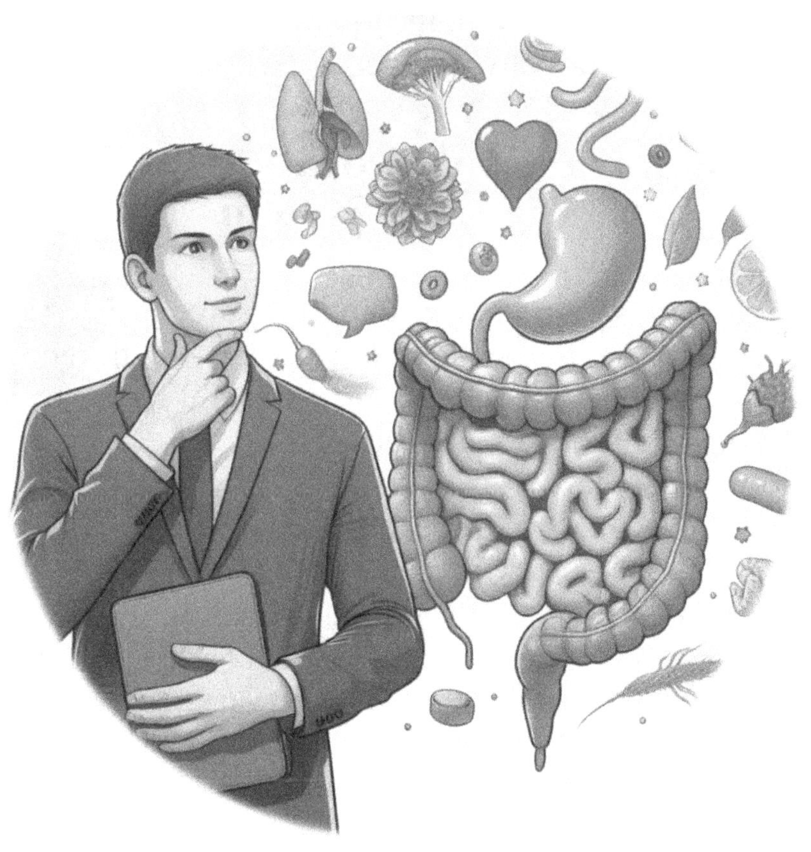

Hydration is often hailed as a cornerstone of good health, but its significance goes beyond quenching thirst or maintaining bodily functions. In this chapter, we'll explore the profound impact hydration has on gut health. From its role in supporting digestion to its influence on gut bacteria, we'll delve into why staying hydrated is crucial for optimal gut function. We'll also discuss how to recognize dehydration, best practices for staying hydrated, foods with high water content, and creative ways to incorporate herbal teas and broths into your daily routine.

Importance of Hydration for the Digestive System

Hydration is essential for supporting proper digestion and ensuring the smooth functioning of the entire gastrointestinal tract. Water plays several key roles in the digestive process, including:

Lubricating the Digestive Tract:

Water helps lubricate the digestive tract, allowing food to move smoothly through the esophagus, stomach, and intestines. Adequate hydration ensures that food is properly broken down and absorbed, preventing issues such as constipation and indigestion.

Facilitating Nutrient Absorption:

Water is necessary for the absorption of nutrients from the digestive tract into the bloodstream. It helps dissolve nutrients, making them more accessible for absorption by the cells lining the intestines. Without proper hydration, nutrient absorption may be impaired, leading to deficiencies and other health issues.

Supporting Waste Elimination:

Water plays a vital role in the formation of stools and the elimination of waste products from the body. Adequate hydration softens stools, making them easier to pass and preventing constipation. It also helps flush toxins and waste materials out of the body, promoting regularity and detoxification.

How Water Affects Gut Bacteria

Proper hydration is not only essential for digestive function but also for maintaining a healthy balance of gut bacteria. The gut microbiota, comprised of trillions of microorganisms, plays a crucial role in digestion, immune function, and overall health. Water influences gut bacteria in several ways:

Maintaining Microbial Balance:

Water helps create an optimal environment for beneficial gut bacteria to thrive. Adequate hydration ensures that the mucosal lining of the intestines remains hydrated, supporting the growth and activity of beneficial microbes while inhibiting the proliferation of harmful bacteria.

Supporting Fermentation:

Water is necessary for the fermentation process that occurs in the colon, where beneficial gut bacteria break down indigestible fibers and produce short-chain fatty acids (SCFAs). These SCFAs provide energy for the cells lining the intestines and help maintain gut health.

Enhancing Immune Function:

Hydration is essential for supporting immune function, which plays a crucial role in maintaining the balance of gut bacteria. A well-hydrated body is better equipped to mount an immune response against harmful pathogens and maintain a healthy balance of gut microbes.

Recognizing Dehydration and Its Effects

Dehydration occurs when the body loses more fluid than it takes in, leading to an imbalance in electrolytes and impaired bodily functions. Recognizing the signs and symptoms of dehydration is essential for maintaining optimal health and preventing complications. Common signs of dehydration include:

- Thirst: Thirst is one of the first indicators of dehydration. When the body's fluid levels are low, the brain signals thirst as a mechanism to prompt fluid intake.

- Dark Urine: Dark-colored urine is a sign of concentrated urine, indicating that the body is trying to conserve water. Inadequate hydration can lead to dark yellow or amber-colored urine.
- Fatigue: Dehydration can cause fatigue and low energy levels as the body struggles to maintain essential functions with limited fluid.
- Dizziness or Lightheadedness: Dehydration can lead to a drop in blood pressure, causing dizziness or lightheadedness, especially when standing up quickly.
- Dry Mouth and Skin: Insufficient hydration can result in dry mouth, lips, and skin as the body conserves moisture for vital functions.

Best Practices for Staying Hydrated

Maintaining proper hydration requires more than just drinking water; it involves adopting healthy habits and mindful practices to support optimal fluid balance. Here are some best practices for staying hydrated:

Drink Plenty of Water:

Make water your beverage of choice throughout the day. Aim to drink at least eight 8-ounce glasses of water daily, or more if you're physically active or live in a hot climate. Carry a reusable water bottle with you to ensure easy access to hydration wherever you go.

Hydrate Regularly:

Establish a routine of drinking water at regular intervals throughout the day. Sip on water consistently rather than waiting until you're thirsty, as thirst is often a late indicator of dehydration.

Monitor Fluid Losses:

Pay attention to factors that increase fluid losses, such as physical activity, hot weather, or illness, and adjust your fluid intake accordingly. Drink extra water to compensate for fluid losses during sweating, urination, or vomiting.

Eat Hydrating Foods:

Incorporate hydrating foods with high water content into your diet, such as fruits, vegetables, soups, and broth-based dishes. These foods not only contribute to your overall fluid intake but also provide essential nutrients and electrolytes.

Limit Dehydrating Beverages:

Reduce your intake of dehydrating beverages such as caffeinated drinks, alcohol, and sugary sodas, which can increase fluid losses and contribute to dehydration. Opt for water, herbal teas, or coconut water as hydrating alternatives.

Listen to Your Body:

Pay attention to your body's thirst signals and respond

promptly by drinking water. Additionally, monitor urine color and frequency as indicators of hydration status. Pale yellow urine is a sign of adequate hydration, while dark-colored urine may indicate dehydration.

Foods with High Water Content

In addition to drinking water, you can boost your fluid intake by consuming foods with high water content. These foods not only provide hydration but also offer essential nutrients, fiber, and antioxidants. Incorporate the following hydrating foods into your diet:

- Cucumbers: Cucumbers are composed of over 95% water, making them an excellent hydrating snack. Enjoy sliced cucumbers on their own, add them to salads, or blend them into refreshing smoothies.

- Watermelon: Watermelon is a delicious and hydrating fruit that contains about 92% water. Enjoy watermelon slices as a refreshing snack, blend them into smoothies, or use them to make hydrating popsicles.

- Oranges: Oranges are rich in water and electrolytes, making them a hydrating choice for replenishing fluids and nutrients. Enjoy fresh oranges as a snack, or squeeze them into juice for a hydrating beverage.

- Strawberries: Strawberries are packed with water and vitamin C, making them a hydrating and nutritious fruit option. Add fresh strawberries to salads, yogurt, or oatmeal for a hydrating boost.

- Tomatoes: Tomatoes are not only hydrating but also rich in antioxidants such as lycopene. Enjoy fresh tomatoes in salads, sandwiches, or salsa for a hydrating and flavorful addition to your meals.

Incorporating Herbal Teas and Broths

In addition to water and hydrating foods, herbal teas and broths can be excellent options for staying hydrated, especially during colder months or when you're looking for a warm and comforting beverage. Herbal teas are caffeine-free and come in a variety of flavors and blends, while broths provide hydration along with electrolytes and minerals. Here are some ways to incorporate herbal teas and broths into your daily routine:

Herbal Teas:

Herbal teas are made from dried herbs, flowers, fruits, or spices and are naturally caffeine-free. They offer a wide range of flavors and health benefits, making them a versatile option for hydration. Enjoy herbal teas hot or cold throughout the day, and experiment with different varieties such as:

- Chamomile: Known for its calming properties, chamomile tea can help promote relaxation and improve sleep quality.

- Peppermint: Peppermint tea is refreshing and soothing to the digestive system, making it an excellent choice after meals or to relieve stomach discomfort.
- Ginger: Ginger tea has anti-inflammatory and digestive benefits, making it a popular choice for soothing nausea and promoting healthy digestion.
- Rooibos: Rooibos tea is rich in antioxidants and has a naturally sweet flavor, making it a delightful option for hydration any time of day.
- Hibiscus: Hibiscus tea is tart and tangy, with vibrant red color and numerous health benefits, including supporting heart health and promoting hydration.

Broths:

Broths are savory liquids made by simmering vegetables, herbs, bones, or meat in water. They are rich in flavor, nutrients, and electrolytes, making them an excellent choice for hydration and nourishment. Enjoy broths as a standalone beverage or use them as a base for soups, stews, and sauces. Consider the following types of broths for hydration:

- Vegetable Broth: Vegetable broth is made by simmering a variety of vegetables, herbs, and spices in water. It's light, flavorful, and packed with vitamins and minerals, making it a nutritious option for hydration.
- Bone Broth: Bone broth is made by simmering animal bones (such as chicken, beef, or fish bones)

in water for an extended period, typically with added vegetables, herbs, and spices. It's rich in collagen, amino acids, and minerals, which support gut health, joint health, and overall well-being.

- Miso Soup: Miso soup is a traditional Japanese dish made with fermented soybean paste (miso), seaweed, tofu, and vegetables. It's flavorful, comforting, and provides hydration along with probiotics and antioxidants.

- Incorporate herbal teas and broths into your daily routine as part of a balanced hydration strategy. Experiment with different flavors and varieties to find ones you enjoy, and sip on them throughout the day to stay hydrated and nourished.

Conclusion

Hydration is essential for supporting optimal gut health and overall well-being. From lubricating the digestive tract to maintaining microbial balance and supporting nutrient absorption, water plays a vital role in digestive function. By staying adequately hydrated and incorporating hydrating foods, herbal teas, and broths into your diet, you can promote hydration, support digestion, and enhance overall health. Pay attention to your body's thirst signals, monitor urine color, and adjust your fluid intake based on activity levels and environmental factors. Remember that staying hydrated is not only about drinking water but also about adopting healthy hydration habits that support your body's needs. By prioritizing hydration and making it a consistent part of your daily routine, you can nourish your body, support gut health, and thrive in all aspects of life.

Part 2:
Gut-Healthy Recipes

Chapter 06

Fiber-Rich Breakfasts

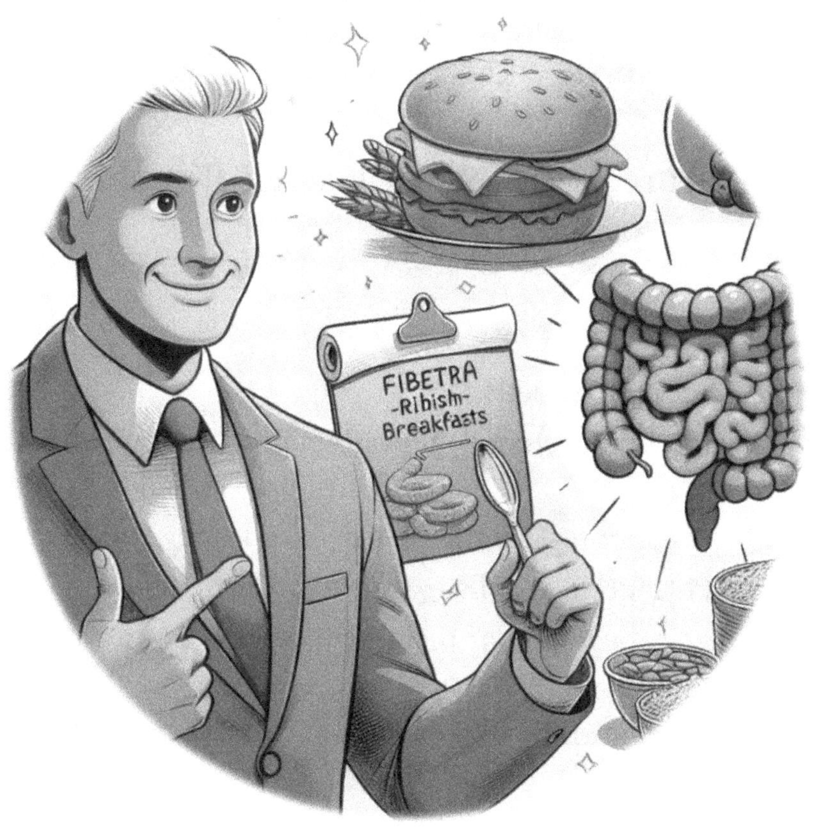

Starting your day with a fiber-rich breakfast sets the tone for healthy digestion and sustained energy throughout the day. In this chapter, we'll explore a variety of delicious and nutritious breakfast options that are packed with fiber to support gut health. From chia seed pudding to veggie-packed omelets, these recipes are not only satisfying and flavorful but also easy to prepare and customizable to suit your tastes and dietary preferences.

Chia Seed Pudding with Berries

Ingredients:

- 1/4 cup chia seeds
- 1 cup unsweetened almond milk (or any milk of choice)
- 1 tablespoon pure maple syrup or honey (optional)
- 1/2 teaspoon vanilla extract
- Fresh berries of choice (e.g., strawberries, blueberries, raspberries)
- Sliced almonds or chopped nuts (optional, for topping)

Instructions:

1. In a bowl or jar, combine chia seeds, almond milk, maple syrup or honey (if using), and vanilla extract. Stir well to combine.

2. Cover the bowl or jar and refrigerate for at least 4 hours or overnight, allowing the chia seeds to absorb the liquid and form a pudding-like consistency.

3. Before serving, give the chia pudding a good stir to redistribute the seeds evenly. Top with fresh berries and sliced almonds or chopped nuts, if desired.

4. Enjoy chilled as a satisfying and fiber-rich breakfast option.

Overnight Oats with Flaxseed and Nuts

Ingredients:

- 1/2 cup rolled oats
- 1 tablespoon ground flaxseed
- 1/2 cup unsweetened almond milk (or any milk of choice)
- 1/2 cup Greek yogurt
- 1 tablespoon pure maple syrup or honey
- 1/2 teaspoon vanilla extract
- Sliced banana or other fruits of choice
- Chopped nuts or seeds (e.g., walnuts, almonds, pumpkin seeds)

Instructions:

1. In a mason jar or container, combine rolled oats, ground flaxseed, almond milk, Greek yogurt, maple syrup or honey, and vanilla extract. Stir well to combine.

2. Add sliced banana or other fruits of choice to the mixture and stir to distribute evenly.

3. Cover the jar or container and refrigerate overnight, allowing the oats to soften and absorb the liquid.

4. In the morning, give the overnight oats a good stir and top with chopped nuts or seeds for added crunch and nutrition.

5. Enjoy cold or at room temperature for a fiber-rich and satisfying breakfast.

High-Fiber Smoothie Bowls

Ingredients:

- 1 frozen banana
- 1/2 cup frozen mixed berries
- 1 cup fresh spinach or kale leaves
- 1 tablespoon chia seeds
- 1 tablespoon ground flaxseed
- 1/2 cup unsweetened almond milk (or any milk of choice)
- Toppings: fresh fruit slices, granola, shredded coconut, nuts or seeds, drizzle of nut butter

Instructions:

1. In a blender, combine frozen banana, frozen mixed berries, fresh spinach or kale leaves, chia seeds, ground flaxseed, and almond milk.

2. Blend until smooth and creamy, adding more almond milk as needed to reach your desired consistency.

3. Pour the smoothie into a bowl and top with your favorite toppings, such as fresh fruit slices, granola, shredded coconut, nuts or seeds, and a drizzle of nut butter.

4. Enjoy with a spoon as a nourishing and fiber-rich breakfast that's as delicious as it is nutritious.

Whole Grain Avocado Toast

Ingredients:

- 2 slices whole grain bread (such as whole wheat or sprouted grain)
- 1 ripe avocado
- Cherry tomatoes, sliced
- Red onion, thinly sliced
- Fresh basil leaves
- Salt and pepper, to taste
- Optional toppings: crumbled feta cheese, hemp seeds, balsamic glaze

Instructions:

1. Toast the whole grain bread slices until golden brown and crispy.

2. While the bread is toasting, mash the ripe avocado in a bowl with a fork until smooth and creamy. Season with salt and pepper to taste.

3. Spread the mashed avocado evenly onto the toasted bread slices.

4. Top the avocado toast with sliced cherry tomatoes, red onion slices, and fresh basil leaves.

5. Sprinkle with additional salt and pepper, and add optional toppings such as crumbled feta cheese, hemp seeds, or a drizzle of balsamic glaze, if desired.

6. Serve immediately and enjoy as a hearty and fiber-rich breakfast option.

Veggie-Packed Omelets

Ingredients:

- 2 large eggs
- 1/4 cup diced bell peppers (any color)
- 1/4 cup diced tomatoes
- 1/4 cup diced mushrooms
- Handful of fresh spinach leaves
- Salt and pepper, to taste
- Cooking oil or butter for greasing the pan
- Optional add-ins: diced onions, chopped broccoli,

grated cheese

Instructions:

1. In a bowl, whisk together the eggs until well beaten. Season with salt and pepper to taste.
2. Heat a non-stick skillet over medium heat and lightly grease with cooking oil or butter.
3. Add diced bell peppers, tomatoes, mushrooms, and any other desired veggies to the skillet. Cook until softened, about 3-4 minutes.
4. Pour the beaten eggs over the cooked vegetables, swirling the pan to distribute evenly.
5. Allow the omelet to cook undisturbed for a few minutes until the edges start to set.
6. Using a spatula, gently lift the edges of the omelet and tilt the skillet to let any uncooked egg mixture flow to the bottom of the pan.
7. Once the omelet is mostly set but still slightly runny on top, sprinkle fresh spinach leaves over one half of the omelet.
8. Carefully fold the other half of the omelet over the spinach to create a half-moon shape. Press down gently with the spatula to seal.
9. Cook for another minute or until the eggs are fully set and the spinach is wilted.
10. Slide the veggie-packed omelet onto a plate and serve hot with a side of whole grain toast or mixed greens for a fiber-rich breakfast.

Yogurt Parfaits with Granola and Fruits

Ingredients:

- Greek yogurt (plain or flavored)
- Homemade or store-bought granola
- Fresh fruits of choice (e.g., berries, sliced bananas, diced mango)
- Optional toppings: honey, maple syrup, shredded coconut, chopped nuts or seeds

Instructions:

1. In a glass or bowl, layer Greek yogurt with granola and fresh fruits of choice.
2. Repeat the layers until the glass or bowl is filled to your liking, alternating between yogurt, granola, and fruits.
3. Drizzle honey or maple syrup over the top for added sweetness, if desired.
4. Sprinkle with shredded coconut, chopped nuts or seeds for extra crunch and nutrition.
5. Serve immediately and enjoy as a refreshing and fiber-rich breakfast parfait.

Conclusion

Incorporating fiber-rich foods into your breakfast routine is a delicious and effective way to support gut health and overall well-being. From chia seed pudding to veggie-packed omelets, these breakfast recipes provide a hearty dose of fiber to keep you feeling satisfied and energized throughout the morning. Whether you prefer sweet or savory options, there's something for everyone to enjoy. Experiment with different ingredients and flavor combinations to create your perfect fiber-rich breakfast and start your day on the right foot.

By incorporating fiber-rich foods into your morning routine, you're not only supporting digestive health but also promoting overall wellness. Fiber helps regulate digestion, stabilize blood sugar levels, and keep you feeling full and satisfied until your next meal. Plus, it nourishes beneficial gut bacteria, which play a crucial role in immune function and nutrient absorption.

Remember to listen to your body and choose breakfast options that make you feel good. Whether you're grabbing a quick smoothie bowl on busy mornings or leisurely enjoying a veggie-packed omelet on the weekend, prioritize fiber-rich foods to support your gut health and well-being.

In the following chapters, we'll continue to explore gut-healthy recipes for every meal of the day, providing you with a variety of delicious and nutritious options to nourish your body and promote optimal digestive function. From satisfying lunches to comforting dinners, you'll find plenty of inspiration to transform your gut health and elevate your culinary repertoire.

Stay tuned as we dive deeper into the world of gut-friendly cuisine and discover how simple, wholesome ingredients can make a significant impact on your health and vitality. Whether you're new to the world of gut health or a seasoned pro, there's always something new to learn and explore on your journey to optimal well-being.

So, grab your apron and get ready to embark on a delicious and nutritious culinary adventure. With these fiber-rich breakfast recipes as your starting point, you'll be well on your way to transforming your gut health and nourishing your body from the inside out. Let's get cooking!

Chapter 07

Nourishing Lunches

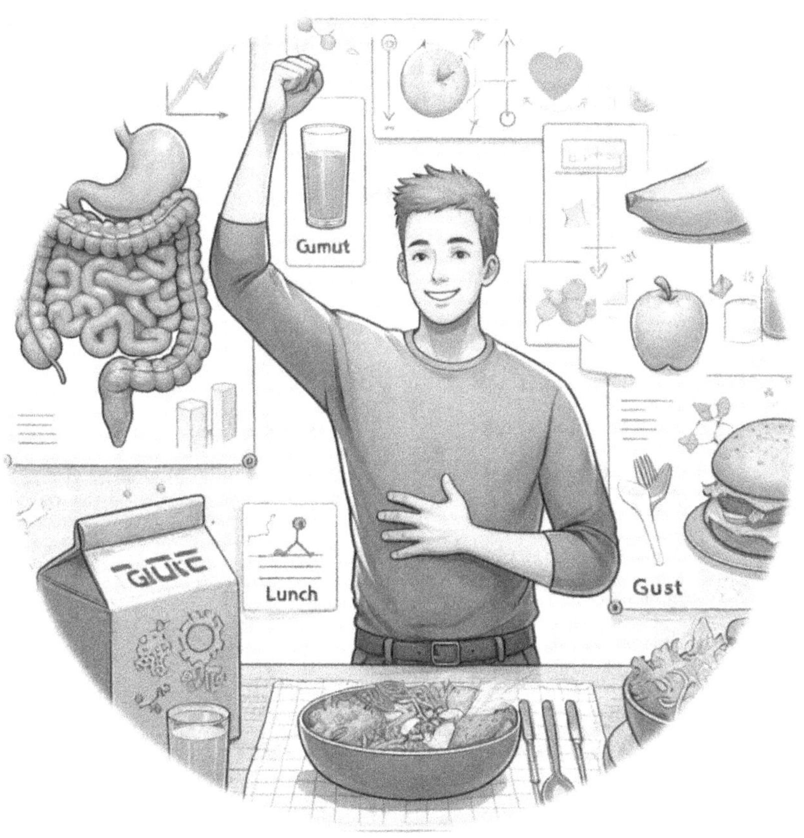

Lunchtime offers an opportunity to refuel your body and nourish it with wholesome ingredients that support gut health. In this chapter, we'll explore a variety of nourishing lunch recipes designed to satisfy your taste buds while providing essential nutrients and fiber to support digestion. From vibrant salads to hearty soups and flavorful wraps, these lunch options are both delicious and gut-friendly, making them perfect for busy weekdays or leisurely weekends.

Quinoa and Black Bean Salad

Ingredients:

- 1 cup cooked quinoa, cooled
- 1 can black beans, drained and rinsed
- 1 cup cherry tomatoes, halved
- 1/2 cup diced bell peppers (any color)
- 1/4 cup chopped cilantro
- 1 avocado, diced
- Juice of 1 lime
- 2 tablespoons olive oil
- Salt and pepper, to taste

Instructions:

1. In a large bowl, combine cooked quinoa, black beans, cherry tomatoes, bell peppers, and chopped cilantro.
2. In a small bowl, whisk together lime juice, olive oil, salt, and pepper to make the dressing.

3. Pour the dressing over the quinoa and black bean mixture and toss gently to coat.

4. Gently fold in diced avocado.

5. Serve chilled or at room temperature as a nourishing and satisfying lunch option.

Lentil Soup with Vegetables

Ingredients:

- 1 cup dried green or brown lentils, rinsed and drained
- 4 cups vegetable broth
- 1 onion, chopped
- 2 carrots, diced
- 2 celery stalks, diced
- 2 cloves garlic, minced
- 1 teaspoon ground cumin
- 1/2 teaspoon ground turmeric
- Salt and pepper, to taste
- Fresh parsley or cilantro, for garnish

Instructions:

1. In a large pot, heat a tablespoon of olive oil over medium heat. Add chopped onion, carrots, and celery, and sauté until softened, about 5 minutes.

2. Add minced garlic, ground cumin, and ground turmeric to the pot, and cook for another minute until fragrant.

3. Add dried lentils and vegetable broth to the pot.

Bring to a boil, then reduce heat and simmer, covered, for 20-25 minutes or until the lentils are tender.

4. Season with salt and pepper to taste.
5. Ladle the lentil soup into bowls and garnish with fresh parsley or cilantro before serving. Enjoy hot as a comforting and nourishing lunch option.

Gut-Friendly Wraps with Fermented Veggies

Ingredients:

- Whole grain or gluten-free wraps
- Hummus or mashed avocado
- Fermented vegetables (e.g., sauerkraut, kimchi)
- Sliced cucumbers
- Shredded carrots
- Fresh spinach or kale leaves
- Sprouts (e.g., alfalfa, broccoli)

Instructions:

1. Lay a whole grain or gluten-free wrap flat on a clean surface.
2. Spread a generous layer of hummus or mashed avocado onto the wrap.
3. Layer fermented vegetables, sliced cucumbers, shredded carrots, fresh spinach or kale leaves, and sprouts on top of the hummus or avocado.
4. Roll up the wrap tightly, folding in the sides as you

go.

5. Slice the wrap in half diagonally and serve immediately, or wrap tightly in parchment paper or foil for later. Enjoy as a convenient and gut-friendly lunch option.

Chickpea and Spinach Curry

Ingredients:

- 1 tablespoon coconut oil or olive oil
- 1 onion, diced
- 2 cloves garlic, minced
- 1 tablespoon grated ginger
- 1 tablespoon curry powder
- 1 teaspoon ground cumin
- 1 teaspoon ground turmeric
- 1 can chickpeas, drained and rinsed
- 1 can diced tomatoes
- 2 cups baby spinach leaves
- 1/2 cup coconut milk
- Salt and pepper, to taste
- Cooked brown rice or quinoa, for serving

Instructions:

1. In a large skillet or pot, heat coconut oil or olive oil over medium heat. Add diced onion and cook until translucent, about 5 minutes.
2. Add minced garlic, grated ginger, curry powder, ground cumin, and ground turmeric to the skillet,

and cook for another minute until fragrant.

3. Stir in chickpeas and diced tomatoes with their juices. Bring to a simmer and cook for 10-15 minutes, allowing the flavors to meld together.

4. Add baby spinach leaves and coconut milk to the skillet, and stir until the spinach wilts and the curry is heated through.

5. Season with salt and pepper to taste.

6. Serve the chickpea and spinach curry over cooked brown rice or quinoa, and garnish with fresh cilantro if desired. Enjoy hot as a flavorful and nourishing lunch option.

Brown Rice Sushi Rolls with Avocado and Cucumber

Ingredients:

- Nori seaweed sheets
- Cooked brown rice
- Avocado, sliced
- Cucumber, julienned
- Carrot, julienned
- Bell pepper, julienned
- Sesame seeds
- Soy sauce or tamari, for dipping
- Pickled ginger and wasabi, optional

Instructions:

1. Place a nori seaweed sheet shiny side down on a

clean surface.

2. Spread a thin layer of cooked brown rice evenly over the nori sheet, leaving a border along the edges.

3. Arrange avocado slices, julienned cucumber, carrot, and bell pepper along the bottom edge of the nori sheet.

4. Sprinkle sesame seeds over the filling.

5. Starting from the bottom edge, tightly roll up the nori sheet, using a bamboo sushi mat or your hands to help shape the roll.

6. Use a sharp knife to slice the sushi roll into bite-sized pieces.

7. Serve the brown rice sushi rolls with soy sauce or tamari for dipping, and optional pickled ginger and wasabi on the side. Enjoy as a nutritious and satisfying lunch option.

Mediterranean Chickpea Salad

Ingredients:

- 1 can chickpeas, drained and rinsed
- 1 cucumber, diced
- 1 bell pepper, diced
- 1/2 red onion, thinly sliced
- 1/4 cup Kalamata olives, pitted and halved
- 1/4 cup crumbled feta cheese (optional)
- Fresh parsley, chopped
- Juice of 1 lemon
- 2 tablespoons extra virgin olive oil

- Salt and pepper, to taste

Instructions:

1. In a large bowl, combine chickpeas, diced cucumber, diced bell pepper, thinly sliced red onion, halved Kalamata olives, and crumbled feta cheese (if using).
2. In a small bowl, whisk together lemon juice, extra virgin olive oil, salt, and pepper to make the dressing.
3. Pour the dressing over the chickpea salad and toss gently to coat.
4. Garnish with fresh chopped parsley before serving.
5. Serve chilled or at room temperature as a refreshing and flavorful lunch option.

Conclusion

These nourishing lunch recipes offer a delightful array of flavors and textures while providing essential nutrients and fiber to support gut health. Whether you're craving a hearty soup, a refreshing salad, or a flavorful wrap, there's something for every palate and dietary preference. By incorporating wholesome ingredients such as legumes, whole grains, vegetables, and fermented foods into your lunchtime meals, you can nourish your body and support optimal digestive function.

From the protein-packed quinoa and black bean salad

to the comforting lentil soup with vegetables, these recipes are designed to keep you feeling satisfied and energized throughout the day. The gut-friendly wraps with fermented veggies offer a convenient and portable option for busy days, while the chickpea and spinach curry provides a flavorful and warming meal that's perfect for cooler weather. For a lighter option, the brown rice sushi rolls with avocado and cucumber offer a refreshing twist on traditional sushi, while the Mediterranean chickpea salad provides a burst of Mediterranean flavors in every bite.

Incorporate these nourishing lunch recipes into your weekly meal rotation to add variety and excitement to your midday meals. Experiment with different ingredients and flavor combinations to create your own unique dishes, and don't be afraid to get creative in the kitchen. Whether you're enjoying lunch at home, at work, or on the go, prioritize nourishing your body with wholesome foods that support gut health and overall well-being.

In the next chapter, we'll explore a variety of satisfying dinner recipes that are both delicious and gut-friendly. From comforting soups and stews to hearty grain bowls and flavorful stir-fries, you'll find plenty of inspiration to elevate your evening meals and nourish your body from within. So, get ready to roll up your sleeves and embark on a culinary adventure that celebrates the power of wholesome ingredients and the joy of nourishing your body with every bite. Let's cook up some delicious dinners that will leave you feeling satisfied, nourished, and ready to take on whatever comes your way.

Chapter 08

Healing Dinners

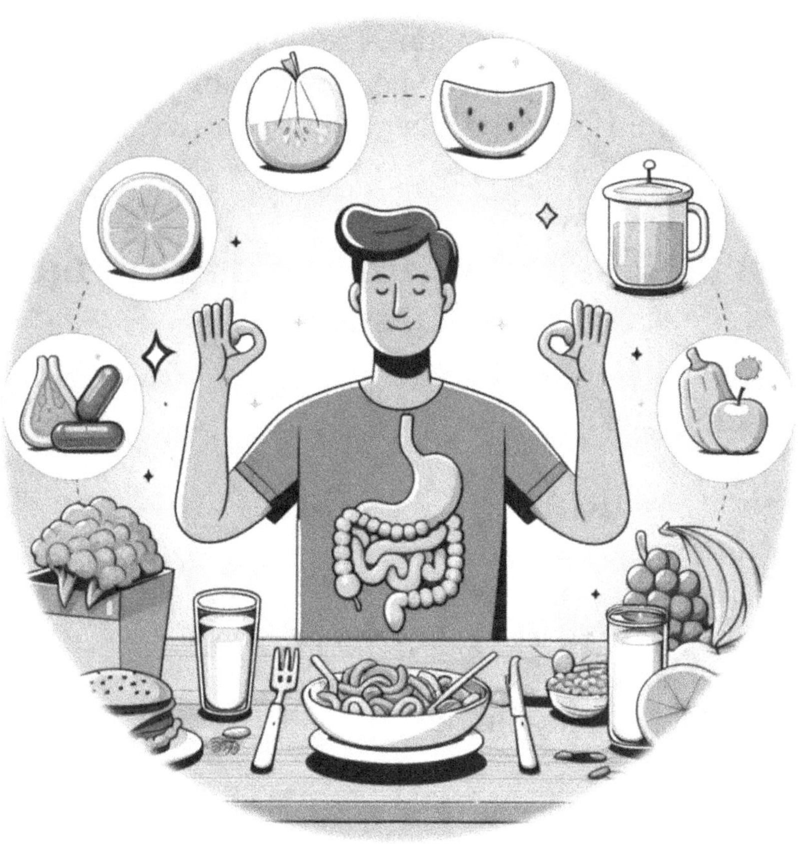

Dinner is the perfect opportunity to wind down from the day and nourish your body with wholesome ingredients that promote healing and well-being. In this chapter, we'll explore a variety of comforting and nutritious dinner recipes designed to support gut health and overall vitality. From protein-rich salmon to hearty vegetarian options, these healing dinners are sure to satisfy your taste buds while providing essential nutrients and fiber to support digestion and promote healing.

Baked Salmon with Asparagus and Quinoa

Ingredients:

- 4 salmon fillets
- 1 bunch asparagus, trimmed
- 1 cup quinoa, rinsed
- 2 cups vegetable broth or water
- 2 tablespoons olive oil
- 2 cloves garlic, minced
- 1 lemon, sliced
- Salt and pepper, to taste
- Fresh herbs (e.g., parsley, dill), for garnish

Instructions:

1. Preheat the oven to 375°F (190°C). Line a baking sheet with parchment paper or lightly grease with olive oil.

2. Place the salmon fillets on one side of the baking sheet and arrange the trimmed asparagus spears on the other side.

3. Drizzle the salmon and asparagus with olive oil and minced garlic. Season with salt and pepper to taste.

4. Place lemon slices on top of the salmon fillets.

5. Bake in the preheated oven for 12-15 minutes, or until the salmon is cooked through and flakes easily with a fork.

6. While the salmon and asparagus are baking, prepare the quinoa. In a saucepan, bring the vegetable broth or water to a boil. Stir in the rinsed quinoa, reduce heat to low, cover, and simmer for 15-20 minutes, or until the quinoa is tender and fluffy.

7. Serve the baked salmon and asparagus alongside the cooked quinoa. Garnish with fresh herbs and lemon wedges, if desired. Enjoy this nourishing and protein-rich dinner option.

Stir-Fried Tofu with Broccoli and Bell Peppers

Ingredients:

- 1 block extra-firm tofu, pressed and cubed
- 2 cups broccoli florets
- 1 bell pepper, thinly sliced
- 2 cloves garlic, minced
- 2 tablespoons soy sauce or tamari

- 1 tablespoon sesame oil
- 1 teaspoon grated ginger
- Cooked brown rice or quinoa, for serving
- Sesame seeds, for garnish

Instructions:

1. Heat sesame oil in a large skillet or wok over medium heat. Add minced garlic and grated ginger, and sauté for 1 minute until fragrant.
2. Add cubed tofu to the skillet and stir-fry until golden brown and crispy on all sides.
3. Add broccoli florets and sliced bell pepper to the skillet, and stir-fry for an additional 3-4 minutes, or until the vegetables are tender-crisp.
4. Stir in soy sauce or tamari, tossing to coat the tofu and vegetables evenly.
5. Serve the stir-fried tofu, broccoli, and bell peppers over cooked brown rice or quinoa. Garnish with sesame seeds before serving. Enjoy this flavorful and plant-based dinner option.

Turmeric Chicken with Sweet Potatoes

Ingredients:

- 4 boneless, skinless chicken breasts
- 2 sweet potatoes, peeled and cubed
- 1 onion, diced
- 2 cloves garlic, minced

- 1 tablespoon olive oil
- 1 teaspoon ground turmeric
- 1/2 teaspoon ground cumin
- 1/2 teaspoon ground paprika
- Salt and pepper, to taste
- Fresh parsley, for garnish

Instructions:

1. Preheat the oven to 400°F (200°C). Line a baking sheet with parchment paper.
2. In a large bowl, toss cubed sweet potatoes with olive oil, minced garlic, ground turmeric, ground cumin, ground paprika, salt, and pepper.
3. Place the seasoned sweet potatoes on one side of the baking sheet.
4. Place the chicken breasts on the other side of the baking sheet. Season the chicken breasts with salt, pepper, and additional ground turmeric if desired.
5. Bake in the preheated oven for 25-30 minutes, or until the chicken is cooked through and the sweet potatoes are tender.
6. Serve the turmeric chicken and sweet potatoes hot, garnished with fresh parsley. Enjoy this wholesome and flavorful dinner option.

Mushroom and Barley Risotto

Ingredients:

- 1 cup pearl barley

- 4 cups vegetable broth
- 2 tablespoons olive oil
- 1 onion, diced
- 2 cloves garlic, minced
- 8 ounces mushrooms (such as cremini or shiitake), sliced
- 1/2 cup dry white wine (optional)
- 1/4 cup grated Parmesan cheese (optional)
- Salt and pepper, to taste
- Fresh parsley, for garnish

Instructions:

1. In a saucepan, bring vegetable broth to a simmer over medium heat. Keep warm while preparing the risotto.
2. In a separate large skillet or pot, heat olive oil over medium heat. Add diced onion and sauté until translucent, about 5 minutes.
3. Add minced garlic and sliced mushrooms to the skillet, and cook until the mushrooms are golden brown and tender, about 8 minutes.
4. Stir in pearl barley and cook for 1-2 minutes, allowing the barley to toast slightly.
5. If using, pour dry white wine into the skillet and stir until absorbed by the barley.
6. Begin adding the warm vegetable broth to the skillet, one ladleful at a time, stirring frequently and allowing the barley to absorb the liquid before adding more.
7. Continue adding broth and stirring until the barley is tender and creamy, about 30-40 minutes.

8. Once the barley is cooked to your desired consistency, remove the skillet from heat.

9. Stir in grated Parmesan cheese, if using, and season with salt and pepper to taste.

10. Serve the mushroom and barley risotto hot, garnished with fresh parsley. Enjoy this comforting and hearty dinner option.

Veggie-Stuffed Bell Peppers

Ingredients:

- 4 bell peppers, tops removed and seeds removed
- 1 cup cooked quinoa or brown rice
- 1 can black beans, drained and rinsed
- 1 cup corn kernels (fresh or frozen)
- 1 cup diced tomatoes
- 1/2 cup diced onion
- 2 cloves garlic, minced
- 1 teaspoon ground cumin
- 1/2 teaspoon chili powder
- Salt and pepper, to taste
- Shredded cheese (such as cheddar or Monterey Jack), for topping
- Fresh cilantro, for garnish

Instructions:

1. Preheat the oven to 375°F (190°C). Grease a baking dish large enough to hold the bell peppers.

2. In a large bowl, combine cooked quinoa or brown

rice, black beans, corn kernels, diced tomatoes, diced onion, minced garlic, ground cumin, chili powder, salt, and pepper.

3. Stuff each bell pepper with the quinoa and vegetable mixture, pressing down gently to pack the filling.

4. Place the stuffed bell peppers upright in the prepared baking dish.

5. Cover the baking dish with aluminum foil and bake in the preheated oven for 25-30 minutes, or until the peppers are tender.

6. Remove the foil and sprinkle shredded cheese on top of each stuffed pepper.

7. Return the peppers to the oven and bake for an additional 5-10 minutes, or until the cheese is melted and bubbly.

8. Serve the veggie-stuffed bell peppers hot, garnished with fresh cilantro. Enjoy this colorful and nutritious dinner option.

Roasted Vegetable Medley

Ingredients:

- Assorted vegetables of choice (e.g., carrots, broccoli, cauliflower, bell peppers, zucchini, cherry tomatoes)
- Olive oil
- Garlic powder
- Dried herbs (e.g., thyme, rosemary, oregano)
- Salt and pepper, to taste

- Balsamic glaze, for serving (optional)

Instructions:

1. Preheat the oven to 400°F (200°C). Line a baking sheet with parchment paper or aluminum foil.
2. Wash and chop the assorted vegetables into bite-sized pieces.
3. Place the chopped vegetables on the prepared baking sheet.
4. Drizzle olive oil over the vegetables and sprinkle with garlic powder, dried herbs, salt, and pepper. Toss until evenly coated.
5. Spread the vegetables out in a single layer on the baking sheet.
6. Roast in the preheated oven for 20-25 minutes, or until the vegetables are tender and lightly browned, stirring halfway through.
7. Remove the roasted vegetables from the oven and transfer to a serving dish.
8. Drizzle with balsamic glaze, if desired, before serving. Enjoy this simple yet flavorful dinner option.

Conclusion

These healing dinner recipes are packed with wholesome ingredients and vibrant flavors to nourish your body and support optimal well-being. From protein-rich salmon to comforting risotto and colorful stuffed bell peppers, there's something for every palate and dietary preference. By incorporating these nutritious and delicious meals into your dinner rotation, you can fuel your body with the nutrients it needs to thrive.

Whether you're cooking for yourself, your family, or guests, these dinner recipes are sure to impress and satisfy. Experiment with different ingredients and flavor combinations to create your own unique dishes, and don't be afraid to get creative in the kitchen. With a focus on fresh, whole foods and simple preparation methods, you can enjoy flavorful and nourishing dinners that support gut health and overall vitality.

In the next section, we'll explore a variety of gut-friendly desserts and snacks to satisfy your sweet tooth and keep you energized between meals. From wholesome snacks to indulgent treats, you'll find plenty of options to curb cravings and promote digestive wellness. So, get ready to satisfy your hunger and nourish your body with these delicious and healing recipes.

Chapter 09

Gut-Boosting Snacks

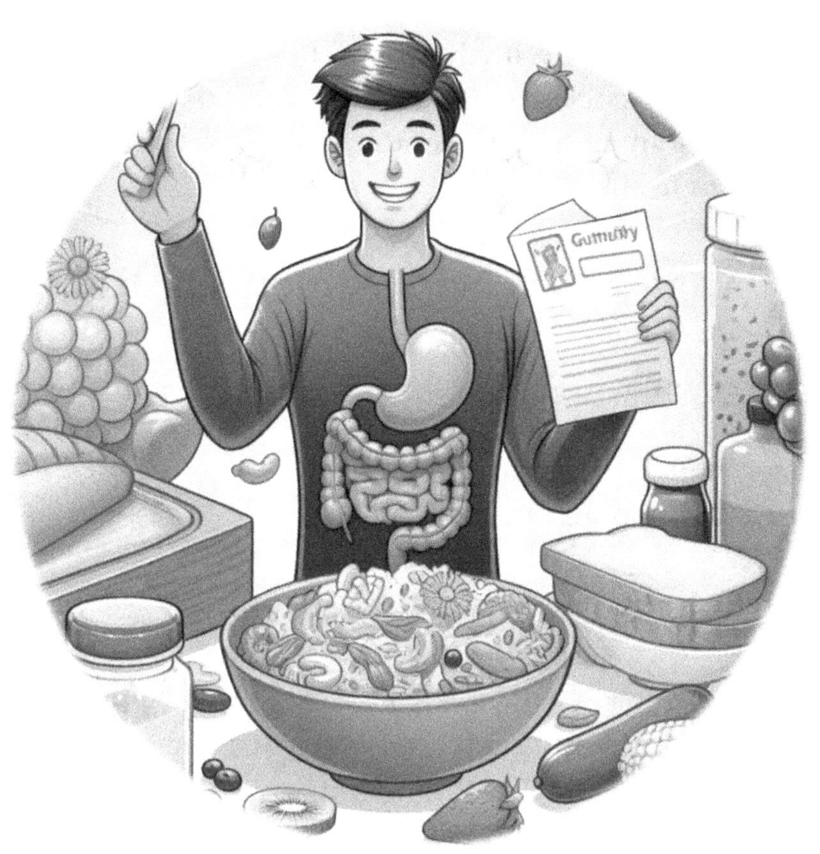

Snacking plays an important role in maintaining energy levels throughout the day while providing an opportunity to nourish your gut with wholesome ingredients. In this chapter, we'll explore a variety of gut-boosting snacks that are not only delicious but also rich in fiber, probiotics, and essential nutrients to support digestive health and overall well-being. From crunchy veggies with hummus to creamy smoothies and energy-packed snacks, these options are perfect for satisfying hunger and promoting gut health between meals.

Apple Slices with Almond Butter

Ingredients:

- 1 apple, cored and sliced
- 2 tablespoons almond butter

Instructions:

1. Core and slice the apple into wedges.
2. Spread almond butter onto each apple slice.
3. Enjoy this simple and satisfying snack that combines the natural sweetness of apples with the creamy richness of almond butter.

Carrot Sticks with Hummus

Ingredients:

- 2 large carrots, peeled and cut into sticks
- 1/4 cup hummus

Instructions:

1. Peel and cut the carrots into sticks.
2. Serve the carrot sticks with hummus for a crunchy and flavorful snack that's packed with fiber and essential nutrients.

Mixed Nuts and Seeds

Ingredients:

- Assorted nuts and seeds (e.g., almonds, walnuts, pumpkin seeds, sunflower seeds)

Instructions:

1. Mix together a variety of nuts and seeds for a nutrient-rich snack that provides a combination of healthy fats, protein, and fiber.
2. Portion out a handful of mixed nuts and seeds for a satisfying and convenient snack on the go.

Fermented Foods like Kimchi and Sauerkraut

Ingredients:

- Fermented vegetables (e.g., kimchi, sauerkraut)

Instructions:

1. Enjoy a serving of fermented vegetables like kimchi or sauerkraut as a gut-friendly snack that's rich in probiotics.
2. Incorporating fermented foods into your diet can help support a healthy balance of gut bacteria and promote digestive wellness.

Smoothie with Kefir and Fruits

Ingredients:

- 1 cup kefir (or yogurt for a dairy-free option)
- Assorted fruits (e.g., berries, banana, mango)
- Handful of spinach or kale leaves
- Optional: chia seeds, flaxseeds, or protein powder

Instructions:

1. In a blender, combine kefir, assorted fruits, and leafy greens.
2. Add optional ingredients like chia seeds, flaxseeds, or protein powder for added nutrition.
3. Blend until smooth and creamy, then pour into a glass and enjoy this refreshing and gut-boosting snack.

Energy Balls with Oats and Chia Seeds

Ingredients:

- 1 cup rolled oats
- 1/2 cup almond butter or peanut butter
- 1/4 cup honey or maple syrup
- 2 tablespoons chia seeds
- Optional mix-ins: dried fruit, chocolate chips, shredded coconut

Instructions:

1. In a large bowl, mix together rolled oats, almond butter or peanut butter, honey or maple syrup, and chia seeds until well combined.
2. Stir in optional mix-ins like dried fruit, chocolate chips, or shredded coconut, if desired.
3. Roll the mixture into bite-sized balls and place them on a baking sheet lined with parchment paper.
4. Refrigerate the energy balls for at least 30 minutes to firm up before serving.
5. Enjoy these wholesome and energy-packed snacks as a convenient option to fuel your body and satisfy hunger between meals.

Conclusion

These gut-boosting snacks are perfect for keeping hunger at bay while nourishing your body with essential nutrients and supporting digestive health. Whether you're craving something sweet, savory, or crunchy, there's a snack option to suit every taste and dietary preference. By incorporating these wholesome snacks into your daily routine, you can promote a healthy balance of gut bacteria and support optimal digestion and overall well-being.

Experiment with different combinations and flavors to keep your snacking routine exciting and satisfying. From simple apple slices with almond butter to nutrient-packed smoothies and energy balls, these snacks are easy to prepare and perfect for enjoying on the go. With a focus on whole, unprocessed foods, you can feel good about nourishing your body with every bite.

In the next section, we'll explore a variety of gut-friendly desserts that satisfy your sweet tooth while providing essential nutrients and promoting digestive wellness. From indulgent treats to lighter options, you'll find plenty of delicious desserts to enjoy guilt-free. So, get ready to satisfy your cravings and support your gut health with these mouthwatering recipes.

Chapter 10

Desserts for Gut Health

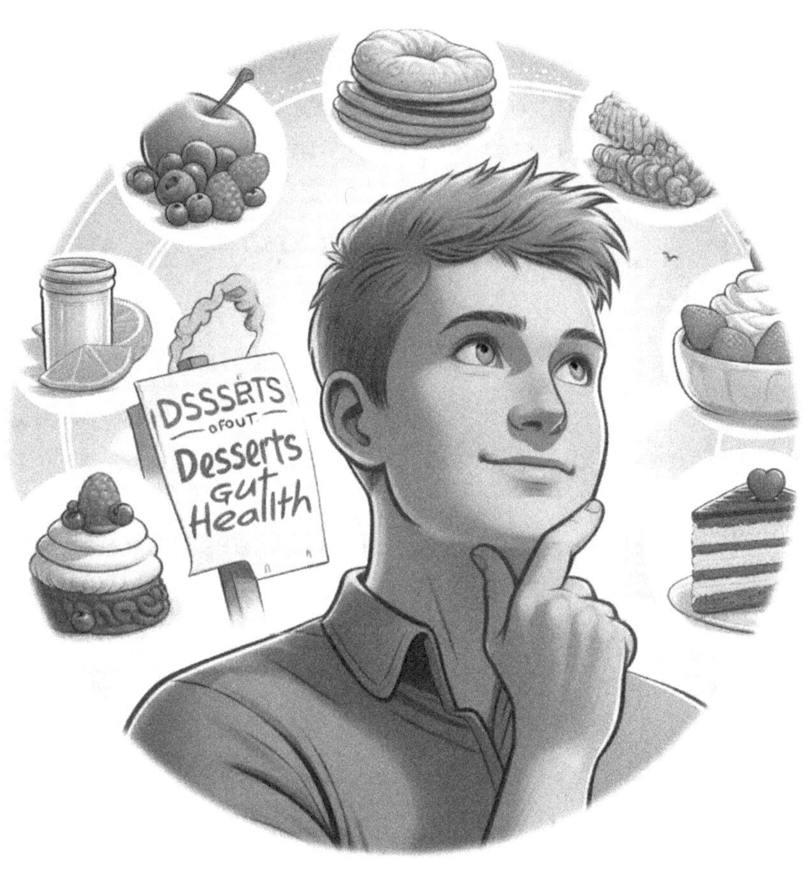

Indulging in desserts doesn't have to mean sacrificing your gut health. In fact, there are plenty of delicious and nutritious dessert options that can actually support digestive wellness. In this chapter, we'll explore a variety of sweet treats that are not only satisfying to the taste buds but also gentle on the digestive system. From antioxidant-rich dark chocolate to fiber-packed fruits and wholesome ingredients like chia seeds and almond flour, these desserts are sure to delight your palate while promoting gut health.

Dark Chocolate and Berry Bark

Ingredients:

- 8 ounces dark chocolate (at least 70% cocoa), chopped
- Assorted berries (e.g., strawberries, blueberries, raspberries)

Instructions:

1. Line a baking sheet with parchment paper.
2. Melt the dark chocolate in a heatproof bowl set over a pot of simmering water, stirring until smooth.
3. Pour the melted chocolate onto the prepared baking sheet and spread it out into an even layer.
4. Arrange the assorted berries on top of the melted chocolate.

5. Place the baking sheet in the refrigerator and chill for at least 30 minutes, or until the chocolate is set.
6. Once set, break the chocolate bark into pieces and serve. Enjoy this antioxidant-rich treat that's perfect for satisfying sweet cravings.

Coconut Yogurt with Pineapple

Ingredients:

- 1 cup coconut yogurt
- 1 cup diced pineapple

Instructions:

1. In a bowl, spoon coconut yogurt.
2. Top with diced pineapple.
3. Enjoy this creamy and tropical dessert that's packed with probiotics and vitamin C.

Chia Seed Pudding with Mango

Ingredients:

- 1/4 cup chia seeds
- 1 cup coconut milk (or any milk of choice)
- 1 tablespoon honey or maple syrup
- 1 ripe mango, diced

Instructions:

1. In a bowl, whisk together chia seeds, coconut milk, and honey or maple syrup.
2. Cover and refrigerate for at least 2 hours, or until the mixture thickens into a pudding-like consistency.
3. Serve the chia seed pudding topped with diced mango for a refreshing and fiber-rich dessert option.

Baked Pears with Cinnamon

Ingredients:

- 4 ripe pears, halved and cored
- 1 tablespoon honey or maple syrup
- 1 teaspoon ground cinnamon
- Optional: chopped nuts or dried fruit for topping

Instructions:

1. Preheat the oven to 375°F (190°C).
2. Place the pear halves cut side up in a baking dish.
3. Drizzle honey or maple syrup over the pears and sprinkle with ground cinnamon.
4. Bake in the preheated oven for 25-30 minutes, or until the pears are tender.
5. Serve the baked pears warm, optionally topped with chopped nuts or dried fruit. Enjoy this

naturally sweet dessert that's rich in fiber and antioxidants.

Almond Flour Brownies

Ingredients:

- 1 1/2 cups almond flour
- 1/4 cup cocoa powder
- 1/2 teaspoon baking soda
- 1/4 teaspoon salt
- 1/2 cup honey or maple syrup
- 1/4 cup melted coconut oil
- 2 eggs
- 1 teaspoon vanilla extract
- Optional: chopped nuts or dark chocolate chunks

Instructions:

1. Preheat the oven to 350°F (175°C). Grease a baking dish or line it with parchment paper.
2. In a large bowl, whisk together almond flour, cocoa powder, baking soda, and salt.
3. In a separate bowl, mix together honey or maple syrup, melted coconut oil, eggs, and vanilla extract.
4. Pour the wet ingredients into the dry ingredients and stir until well combined.
5. Fold in optional chopped nuts or dark chocolate chunks, if desired.
6. Pour the batter into the prepared baking dish and

spread it out into an even layer.

7. Bake in the preheated oven for 20-25 minutes, or until a toothpick inserted into the center comes out clean.

8. Allow the brownies to cool before slicing and serving. Enjoy these moist and fudgy brownies made with wholesome almond flour.

Blueberry Oat Bars

Ingredients:

- 2 cups rolled oats
- 1 cup almond flour
- 1/4 cup honey or maple syrup
- 1/4 cup melted coconut oil
- 1 teaspoon vanilla extract
- 1 cup fresh or frozen blueberries

Instructions:

1. Preheat the oven to 350°F (175°C). Grease a baking dish or line it with parchment paper.

2. In a large bowl, combine rolled oats, almond flour, honey or maple syrup, melted coconut oil, and vanilla extract. Mix until well combined.

3. Press half of the oat mixture into the bottom of the prepared baking dish.

4. Spread the blueberries evenly over the oat mixture.

5. Crumble the remaining oat mixture over the top of

the blueberries.

6. Bake in the preheated oven for 30-35 minutes, or until the top is golden brown.

7. Allow the blueberry oat bars to cool before slicing into squares. Enjoy these wholesome and fruity bars as a satisfying dessert or snack option.

Conclusion

These desserts for gut health offer a delightful way to satisfy your sweet tooth while nourishing your body with wholesome ingredients. From antioxidant-rich dark chocolate and berry bark to creamy coconut yogurt with pineapple and fiber-packed chia seed pudding with mango, there's something for every craving and dietary preference. By incorporating these nutritious and delicious desserts into your routine, you can support digestive wellness and indulge in guilt-free treats that leave you feeling satisfied and energized.

Experiment with different flavor combinations and ingredients to create your own unique desserts that cater to your taste preferences. Whether you're enjoying a simple fruit-based dessert or indulging in a decadent brownie or bar, these recipes are easy to prepare and perfect for sharing with family and friends. With a focus on whole, unprocessed foods and natural sweeteners, you can feel good about treating yourself to these gut-friendly desserts that support optimal well-being.

Part 3:
Advanced Strategies and Lifestyle Tips

Chapter 11

Probiotics and Prebiotics

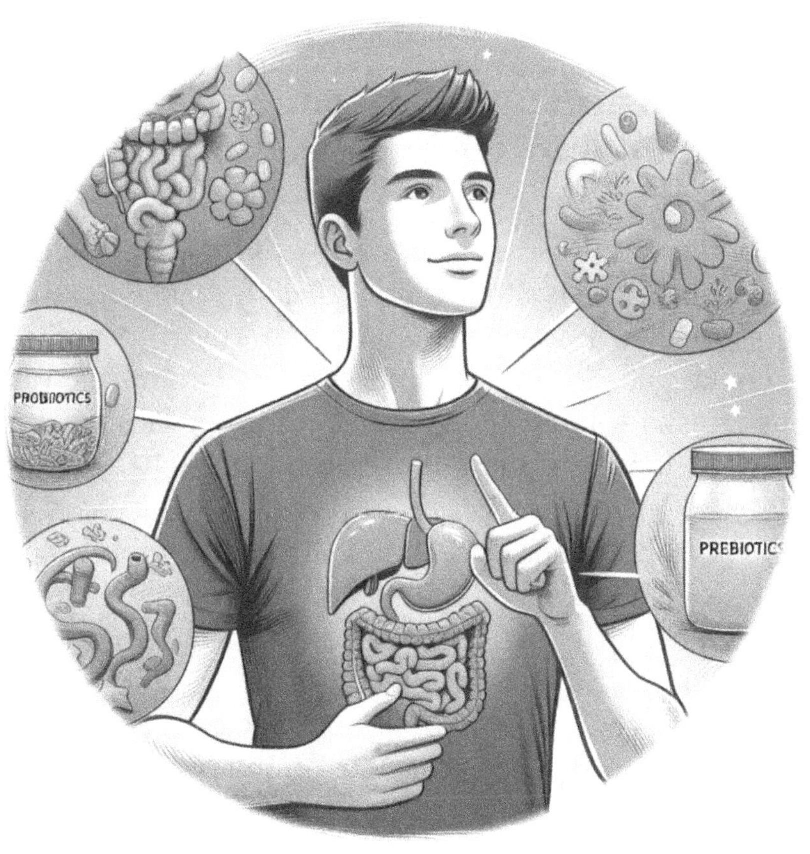

In the quest for optimal gut health, understanding the role of probiotics and prebiotics is essential. These dynamic duo components play a crucial role in fostering a healthy gut environment, promoting digestion, and bolstering overall well-being. In this chapter, we'll delve into the definitions, sources, benefits, and strategies for incorporating probiotics and prebiotics into your diet for a thriving gut ecosystem.

Definition and Difference between Probiotics and Prebiotics

Probiotics are live microorganisms, primarily bacteria and some yeasts, that confer health benefits when consumed in adequate amounts. These beneficial bacteria colonize the gut and support various aspects of digestive health, including nutrient absorption, immune function, and gut barrier integrity.

On the other hand, prebiotics are indigestible fibers that serve as food for probiotics, helping them thrive and multiply in the gut. Prebiotics pass through the digestive tract intact until they reach the colon, where they undergo fermentation by gut bacteria, producing short-chain fatty acids that nourish the colon cells and contribute to overall gut health.

Natural Sources of Probiotics

Incorporating probiotic-rich foods into your diet is an excellent way to promote a healthy gut microbiome.

Some natural sources of probiotics include:

- Yogurt: Fermented dairy product containing live cultures of bacteria, such as Lactobacillus and Bifidobacterium.
- Kefir: Fermented milk drink made from kefir grains, containing a diverse array of beneficial bacteria and yeasts.
- Sauerkraut: Fermented cabbage rich in probiotics, particularly Lactobacillus bacteria.
- Kimchi: Traditional Korean fermented dish made from vegetables, including cabbage and radishes, seasoned with spices and probiotic-rich microbes.

Foods Rich in Prebiotics

Incorporating prebiotic-rich foods into your diet provides nourishment for beneficial gut bacteria. Some foods rich in prebiotics include:

- Garlic: Contains prebiotic fibers, particularly fructooligosaccharides (FOS), that support the growth of beneficial bacteria in the gut.
- Onions: Rich in inulin, a type of prebiotic fiber that promotes the proliferation of probiotic bacteria.
- Bananas: Source of resistant starch, a prebiotic fiber that fuels the growth of beneficial gut bacteria and supports digestive health.
- Asparagus: Contains inulin and other prebiotic fibers that stimulate the growth of beneficial bacteria in the gut.

Benefits of Combining Probiotics and Prebiotics

Consuming both probiotics and prebiotics in tandem can have synergistic effects on gut health. Prebiotics serve as fuel for probiotics, enhancing their survival and activity in the gut. This symbiotic relationship between probiotics and prebiotics promotes a balanced gut microbiome, supports digestion, strengthens the immune system, and may reduce the risk of digestive disorders such as irritable bowel syndrome (IBS) and inflammatory bowel disease (IBD).

How to Choose Probiotic Supplements

When selecting probiotic supplements, it's essential to consider several factors to ensure efficacy and safety:

- Strain Diversity: Look for supplements containing multiple strains of probiotic bacteria, including Lactobacillus and Bifidobacterium species, to target different areas of the gut and maximize benefits.
- Viable Cells: Choose supplements with a high number of viable cells (colony-forming units, or CFUs) at the time of expiration to ensure potency and efficacy.
- Stability: Opt for supplements that are shelf-stable and resistant to stomach acid, ensuring survival and delivery of probiotic bacteria to the intestines.

Tips for Incorporating Probiotics and Prebiotics into Daily Meals

Integrating probiotics and prebiotics into your daily meals doesn't have to be complicated. Here are some practical tips:

- Enjoy Fermented Foods: Incorporate probiotic-rich foods like yogurt, kefir, sauerkraut, and kimchi into your meals or snacks.
- Add Prebiotic Foods: Include prebiotic-rich foods such as garlic, onions, bananas, and asparagus in your salads, stir-fries, soups, or side dishes.
- Blend Smoothies: Prepare smoothies with yogurt or kefir as the base and add fruits like bananas or berries, along with leafy greens like spinach or kale for added prebiotic fiber.
- Top with Fiber: Sprinkle ground flaxseeds, chia seeds, or oats onto yogurt or oatmeal for an extra dose of prebiotic fiber.
- Experiment with Recipes: Get creative in the kitchen by experimenting with probiotic and prebiotic ingredients in your favorite recipes, such as yogurt-based dips, fermented vegetable salads, or whole grain dishes.

By incorporating probiotics and prebiotics into your diet through a variety of foods and supplements, you can support a diverse and balanced gut microbiome, enhance digestive health, and promote overall well-being. Experiment with different sources and combinations to find what works best for you and enjoy the benefits of a thriving gut ecosystem.

Chapter 12

Managing Stress for a Healthier Gut

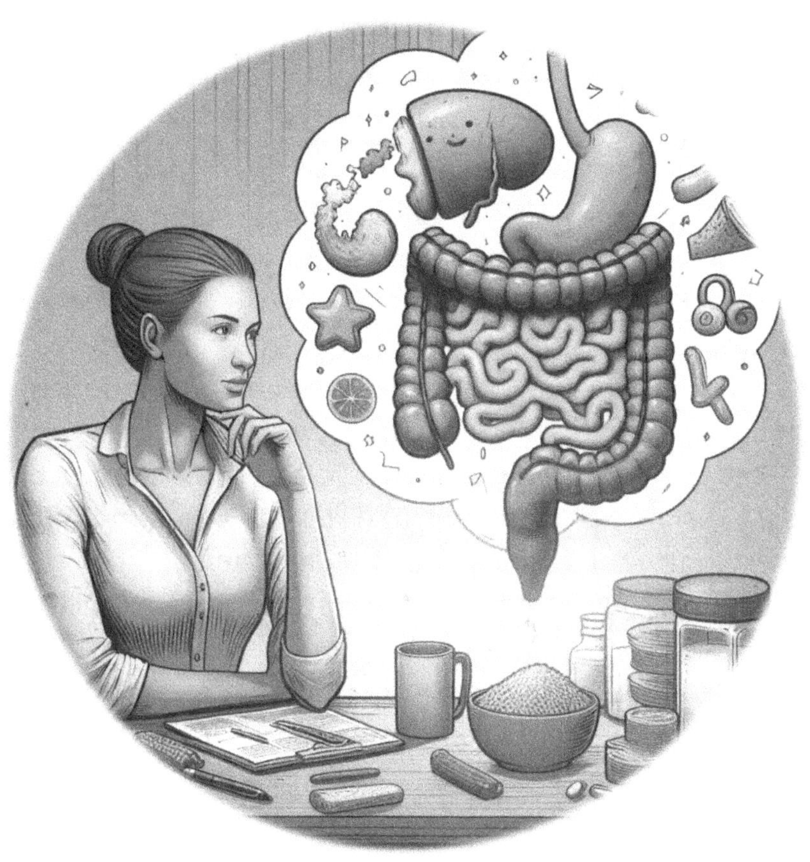

In the hustle and bustle of modern life, stress has become an unavoidable companion for many. However, its impact extends far beyond mere mental tension, permeating into every aspect of our well-being, including gut health. In this chapter, we'll explore the intricate connection between stress and gut health, as well as practical strategies for managing stress to promote a healthier gut and overall vitality.

Understanding the Stress-Gut Health Connection

The gut-brain axis, a bidirectional communication network between the gut and the brain, serves as a conduit for the profound influence of stress on gastrointestinal function. When you experience stress, whether it's due to work pressures, relationship challenges, or financial worries, your body initiates a cascade of physiological responses, including the release of stress hormones like cortisol and adrenaline. These hormones can disrupt the delicate balance of the gut microbiota, compromise intestinal barrier function, and exacerbate inflammation in the gastrointestinal tract, leading to digestive discomfort, irregular bowel movements, and exacerbation of gastrointestinal conditions such as irritable bowel syndrome (IBS) and inflammatory bowel disease (IBD).

Stress Reduction Techniques for Gut Health

Mindfulness Meditation

Mindfulness meditation, a practice rooted in ancient contemplative traditions, offers a powerful antidote to stress and cultivates a sense of calm and clarity amidst life's challenges. By focusing on the present moment without judgment, you can cultivate awareness of your thoughts, emotions, and bodily sensations, allowing you to respond to stressors with greater equanimity and resilience. Incorporate mindfulness meditation into your daily routine by setting aside a few minutes each day to sit quietly, observe your breath, and tune into the sensations in your body. Over time, this practice can help reduce stress-related symptoms and promote gut health by modulating the stress response and promoting relaxation.

Yoga Practice

Yoga, an ancient discipline that integrates physical postures, breathwork, and meditation, offers a holistic approach to stress management and gut health. Through the practice of asanas (yoga poses) and pranayama (breath control), you can release tension from the body, quiet the mind, and promote a sense of balance and well-being. Incorporate gentle yoga sequences into your daily routine to stretch and strengthen your body, alleviate muscular tension, and enhance digestive function. Focus on deep, diaphragmatic breathing to stimulate the parasympathetic nervous system, which promotes relaxation and digestion. Whether you prefer a restorative yin yoga practice or an invigorating vinyasa flow, find a style of yoga that resonates with you and commit to regular practice for optimal stress relief and gut health.

Regular Exercise

Regular physical activity is a potent stress-buster and a cornerstone of a healthy lifestyle. Engaging in aerobic exercise, strength training, or mind-body activities like tai chi or qigong can help alleviate stress, boost mood, and promote overall well-being. Exercise stimulates the release of endorphins, neurotransmitters that act as natural painkillers and mood elevators, helping to reduce stress and promote feelings of happiness and relaxation. Aim for at least 30 minutes of moderate-intensity exercise most days of the week to reap the stress-reducing benefits and support gut health. Whether you enjoy brisk walking, cycling, swimming, or dancing, find activities that you enjoy and incorporate them into your daily routine for optimal stress management and digestive wellness.

Importance of Adequate Sleep

Inadequate sleep is a common consequence of chronic stress, yet it can further exacerbate stress levels and compromise gut health. Sleep plays a crucial role in regulating stress hormones, supporting immune function, and facilitating tissue repair and regeneration, including the repair of the intestinal mucosa. When you're sleep-deprived, your body produces more stress hormones like cortisol, which can disrupt the balance of the gut microbiota, increase intestinal permeability, and exacerbate gastrointestinal inflammation. Prioritize sleep hygiene by creating a relaxing bedtime routine, establishing a consistent sleep schedule, and optimizing your sleep environment for restorative rest. Aim for 7-9 hours of quality sleep per night to support optimal stress management and gut health.

Breathing Exercises for Digestion

Deep breathing exercises offer a simple yet effective way to calm the mind, relax the body, and promote optimal digestion. By practicing deep, diaphragmatic breathing, you can activate the parasympathetic nervous system, also known as the "rest and digest" response, which promotes relaxation and enhances digestive function. Incorporate breathing exercises into your daily routine to support gut health and reduce stress levels. Try the following technique:

Abdominal Breathing Technique

1. Find a comfortable seated position or lie down on your back.
2. Place one hand on your chest and the other hand on your abdomen.
3. Inhale deeply through your nose, allowing your abdomen to rise as you fill your lungs with air.
4. Exhale slowly and completely through your mouth, drawing your navel toward your spine to expel the

air.

5. Continue to breathe deeply and rhythmically, focusing on the sensation of your breath moving in and out of your body.

6. Practice this breathing technique for 5-10 minutes, gradually increasing the duration as you become more comfortable with the practice.

Creating a Relaxing Eating Environment

- The way you eat can also impact your digestion and stress levels. Creating a relaxing eating environment can help promote mindful eating and optimal digestion. Here are some tips for creating a calming atmosphere during meals:

- Mindful Eating: Take time to savor each bite, chewing slowly and paying attention to the flavors, textures, and sensations of the food. Avoid distractions such as electronic devices or stressful conversations, and focus on the act of eating. Engage your senses by appreciating the aroma, appearance, and taste of your meals, fostering a deeper connection with your food and promoting satiety.

- Reduce Distractions: Create a peaceful dining environment free from distractions such as television, phones, or work-related activities. Set aside dedicated time for meals and focus on enjoying the nourishing experience of eating without external interruptions.

- Mind-Body Connection: Practice gratitude and mindfulness before meals to cultivate a sense of appreciation and presence. Take a few moments to express gratitude for the nourishing food on your plate and the opportunity to nourish your body and soul.

- Optimal Posture: Maintain good posture while eating to support optimal digestion and reduce discomfort. Sit upright with your shoulders relaxed and your spine aligned, allowing for proper alignment of the digestive organs and efficient food transit through the gastrointestinal tract.

- Chew Thoroughly: Take the time to chew your food thoroughly, breaking it down into smaller particles and initiating the digestive process. Chewing stimulates the release of saliva, which contains digestive enzymes that begin the breakdown of carbohydrates and fats in the mouth, facilitating efficient digestion and nutrient absorption.

- Practice Gratitude: Cultivate an attitude of gratitude and appreciation for the nourishing food on your plate and the abundance of blessings in your life. Reflect on the journey of your food from farm to table, acknowledging the efforts of farmers, producers, and all beings involved in the food production process.

By creating a relaxing eating environment and practicing mindfulness during meals, you can enhance digestion, reduce stress, and promote overall well-being.

Long-Term Stress Management Strategies

In addition to incorporating stress reduction techniques into your daily routine, it's essential to adopt long-term stress management strategies to support gut health and overall vitality. Here are some additional strategies to consider:

- Establish Healthy Boundaries: Set boundaries and prioritize self-care to prevent burnout and overwhelm. Learn to say no to commitments that don't align with your values or contribute to your well-being, and make time for activities that bring you joy and relaxation.

- Cultivate Resilience: Cultivate resilience by reframing challenges as opportunities for growth and learning. Practice positive self-talk, resilience-building exercises, and gratitude journaling to cultivate a resilient mindset and navigate life's ups and downs with grace and resilience.

- Seek Support: Reach out for support from friends, family, or mental health professionals if you're feeling overwhelmed or struggling to cope with stress. Surround yourself with a supportive network of individuals who uplift and encourage you, and don't hesitate to ask for help when needed.

- Prioritize Self-Care: Make self-care a non-negotiable priority in your life, prioritizing activities that nourish your body, mind, and soul. Engage in activities that bring you joy, whether it's spending time in nature, practicing creative expression, or indulging in a soothing bath or massage.

- Practice Gratitude: Cultivate an attitude of gratitude by regularly expressing appreciation for the blessings in your life. Keep a gratitude journal, write thank-you notes, or simply take a moment each day to reflect on the things you're grateful for, fostering a sense of abundance and contentment.

- Stay Active: Regular physical activity is a powerful antidote to stress, promoting the release of endorphins and enhancing mood and well-being. Find activities that you enjoy and incorporate them into your daily routine, whether it's walking, dancing, cycling, or practicing yoga.

By adopting these long-term stress management strategies, you can cultivate resilience, reduce stress levels, and support gut health for optimal vitality and well-being.

Conclusion

Managing stress is essential for maintaining optimal gut health and overall well-being. By understanding the connection between stress and gut health and incorporating stress reduction techniques into your daily routine, you can support digestive wellness and promote a balanced and resilient gut microbiome. Whether it's practicing mindfulness, engaging in regular exercise, prioritizing sleep, or creating a relaxing eating environment, there are countless ways to manage stress and support gut health. By prioritizing self-care, cultivating resilience, and seeking support when needed, you can navigate life's challenges with grace and resilience, fostering a healthier gut and a happier life.

Chapter 13

Exercise and Gut Health

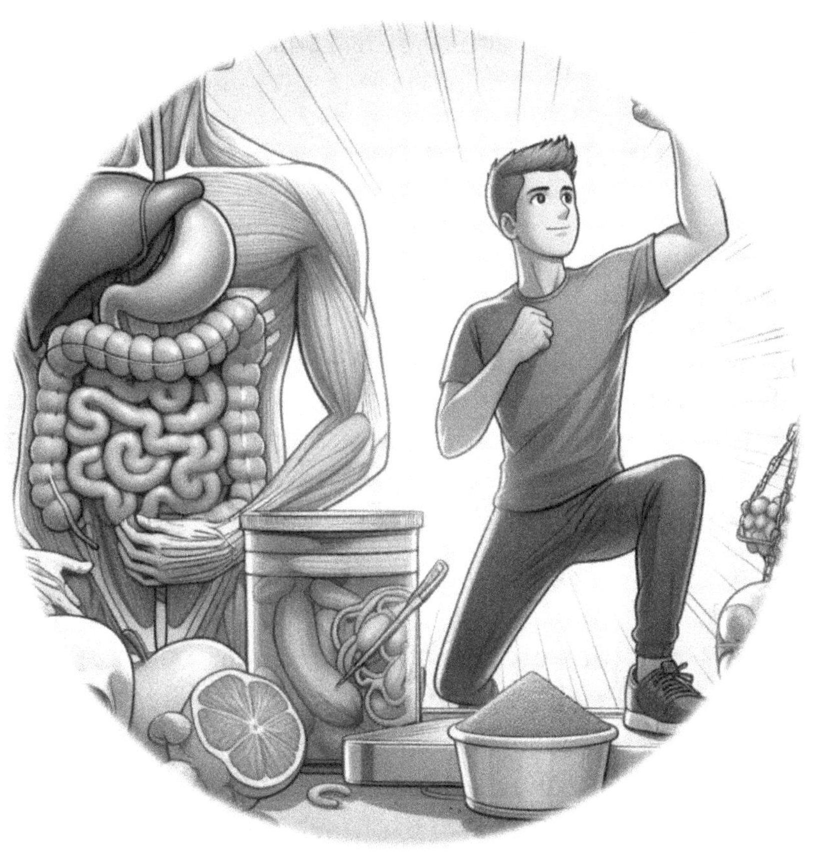

Physical activity isn't just about building muscle or improving cardiovascular health—it also plays a crucial role in maintaining a healthy gut. In this chapter, we'll explore how exercise benefits the digestive system, the types of exercises most beneficial for gut health, strategies for creating a balanced workout routine, the importance of consistency, and how to integrate movement into your daily life. We'll also discuss hydration and nutrition tips to support the unique needs of active individuals.

Understanding the Gut-Exercise Connection

The relationship between exercise and gut health is multifaceted, with physical activity exerting positive effects on various aspects of digestive function. Regular exercise promotes motility in the gastrointestinal tract, helping to prevent constipation and alleviate symptoms of digestive discomfort. Additionally, exercise has been shown to modulate the composition and diversity of the gut microbiota, promoting the growth of beneficial bacteria and reducing the risk of gastrointestinal disorders such as inflammatory bowel disease (IBD) and irritable bowel syndrome (IBS). Furthermore, exercise helps regulate stress hormones like cortisol, which can impact gut function and exacerbate digestive symptoms.

Types of Exercise Most Beneficial for Gut Health

While any form of physical activity can benefit gut health, certain types of exercise have been shown to have particularly positive effects on digestive function. Here are some examples:

Aerobic Exercise

Aerobic exercise, also known as cardiovascular exercise, stimulates blood flow to the digestive organs and promotes peristalsis, the wave-like contractions that move food through the digestive tract. Activities like brisk walking, jogging, cycling, swimming, and dancing can help improve digestion and alleviate symptoms of gastrointestinal discomfort.

Resistance Training

Resistance training, or strength training, helps build muscle mass and increase metabolic rate, which can have indirect benefits for gut health. By improving overall metabolic function and insulin sensitivity, resistance training may help regulate blood sugar levels and reduce the risk of metabolic disorders that can impact digestive health.

Yoga and Pilates

Yoga and Pilates offer gentle yet effective forms of exercise that focus on improving flexibility, strength, and body awareness. These mind-body practices incorporate breathwork and movement sequences that stimulate digestion, reduce stress, and promote relaxation, making them ideal for supporting gut health.

Creating a Balanced Workout Routine

To reap the full benefits of exercise for gut health, it's important to create a balanced workout routine that includes a variety of activities to target different aspects of fitness. Here are some tips for designing a well-rounded exercise program:

Include Aerobic Exercise

Incorporate aerobic exercise into your routine at least three to five times per week, aiming for a total of 150 minutes of moderate-intensity activity or 75 minutes of vigorous-intensity activity per week. Choose activities that you enjoy and can sustain for an extended period, such as walking, jogging, cycling, or swimming.

Incorporate Resistance Training

Integrate resistance training exercises into your routine

two to three times per week, focusing on major muscle groups such as the legs, arms, back, and core. Use a combination of bodyweight exercises, free weights, resistance bands, or weight machines to challenge your muscles and promote strength and endurance.

Prioritize Flexibility and Mobility

Include flexibility and mobility exercises in your routine to improve joint range of motion, prevent injury, and enhance overall movement quality. Incorporate dynamic stretches, static stretches, and mobility drills that target key areas of tightness or stiffness, such as the hips, shoulders, and spine.

Mix It Up

Avoid monotony by varying your workouts and trying new activities to keep your body and mind engaged. Experiment with different types of exercise, such as yoga, Pilates, dance, hiking, or martial arts, to discover what you enjoy and what works best for your body.

Listen to Your Body

Pay attention to your body's signals and adjust your workouts accordingly. If you're feeling fatigued or sore, give yourself permission to take a rest day or engage in gentle, low-impact activities like stretching or walking. Be mindful of any pain or discomfort and consult with a healthcare professional if you experience persistent or severe symptoms.

Importance of Consistency

Consistency is key when it comes to reaping the benefits of exercise for gut health. Make physical activity a regular part of your routine by scheduling workouts at the same time each day or week and prioritizing movement as an essential aspect of self-care. Set realistic goals and gradually increase the duration, intensity, and frequency of your workouts over time to avoid burnout and sustain long-term adherence.

Integrating Movement into Daily Life

In addition to structured exercise sessions, look for opportunities to incorporate movement into your daily life to support gut health and overall well-being. Here are some simple strategies to get moving throughout the day:

Take Active Breaks

Break up long periods of sitting or sedentary activity by taking short active breaks to stretch, walk, or move around. Set a timer to remind yourself to stand up, stretch your muscles, and take a brief walk around your home or office every hour.

Walk Whenever Possible

Choose walking as your primary mode of transportation whenever feasible. Instead of driving or taking public transit, opt to walk or bike to nearby destinations to increase your daily step count and enjoy the health benefits of physical activity.

Use Movement-Friendly Tools

Incorporate movement-friendly tools and equipment into your daily routine to encourage active living. Invest in a standing desk or adjustable workstation to alternate between sitting and standing throughout the day. Use a stability ball or active sitting cushion to engage your core muscles while sitting at your desk.

Engage in Household Chores

Turn household chores into opportunities for physical activity by tackling tasks like cleaning, gardening, or yard work. Sweep, vacuum, mop, or dust your home to get your heart pumping and burn calories while maintaining a tidy living space.

Practice Active Leisure

Choose recreational activities that involve movement and physical exertion, such as hiking, dancing, playing sports, or practicing outdoor activities like gardening, birdwatching, or photography. Invite friends or family to join you for active outings and enjoy the social and physical benefits of shared experiences.

Hydration and Nutrition Tips for Active Individuals

Staying hydrated and nourished is essential for supporting optimal performance during exercise and promoting recovery afterward. Here are some hydration and nutrition tips for active individuals:

Drink Plenty of Water

Stay hydrated before, during, and after exercise by drinking water regularly throughout the day. Aim to consume at least 8-10 cups of water per day, or more if you're engaging in intense or prolonged physical activity.

Replenish Electrolytes

Replace electrolytes lost through sweat by consuming sports drinks or electrolyte-enhanced beverages during prolonged or intense exercise sessions. Alternatively, incorporate electrolyte-rich foods such as bananas, oranges, coconut water, or broth into your post-workout meals and snacks.

Eat a Balanced Diet

Fuel your body with a balanced diet rich in nutrient-dense foods to support energy production, muscle repair, and recovery. Focus on consuming a variety of whole foods, including lean proteins, complex carbohydrates, healthy fats, fruits, and vegetables, to provide the essential nutrients your body needs to perform optimally. Prioritize nutrient timing by consuming a balanced meal or snack containing carbohydrates and protein within 30-60 minutes post-exercise to replenish glycogen stores and support muscle repair and growth.

Snack Smart

Choose nutrient-rich snacks to fuel your workouts and curb hunger between meals. Opt for portable options like trail mix, Greek yogurt with fruit, whole grain crackers with nut butter, or veggie sticks with hummus to provide sustained energy and promote recovery.

Listen to Your Hunger Cues

Pay attention to your body's hunger and satiety signals and fuel accordingly. Eat when you're hungry and stop when you're satisfied, honoring your body's natural cues for nourishment and replenishment.

Plan Ahead

Plan and prepare nutritious meals and snacks in advance to ensure you have healthy options readily available when hunger strikes. Batch cook staples like grains, proteins, and vegetables to assemble quick and convenient meals throughout the week.

Monitor Hydration Status

Monitor your hydration status by paying attention to thirst cues, urine color, and sweat rate during exercise. Drink fluids regularly to maintain hydration levels and prevent dehydration, particularly in hot or humid conditions.

Choose Whole Foods

Prioritize whole, minimally processed foods over highly processed or refined options to maximize nutrient intake and support overall health. Choose whole grains, lean proteins, healthy fats, fruits, and vegetables as the foundation of your diet to provide essential vitamins, minerals, fiber, and antioxidants.

Experiment with Timing

Experiment with meal timing and composition to optimize performance and recovery based on your individual preferences and needs. Some athletes may benefit from consuming a small snack or carbohydrate-rich meal 30-60 minutes before exercise to provide immediate energy, while others may prefer to exercise in a fasted state and refuel afterward.

Stay Flexible

Be flexible with your nutrition plan and adjust it based on your changing schedule, preferences, and goals. Focus on consistency and balance rather than perfection, and allow yourself the flexibility to enjoy occasional treats or indulgences without guilt.

By following these hydration and nutrition tips for active individuals, you can support optimal performance, promote recovery, and enhance overall health and well-being.

Conclusion

Exercise plays a crucial role in supporting gut health and overall well-being. By incorporating regular physical activity into your routine, you can improve digestive function, reduce stress, and support a balanced gut microbiome. Whether you prefer aerobic exercise, resistance training, yoga, or Pilates, finding activities that you enjoy and can sustain long-term is key to reaping the benefits of exercise for gut health. By staying consistent, listening to your body, and prioritizing hydration and nutrition, you can cultivate a healthy lifestyle that supports digestive wellness and vitality for years to come.

Chapter 14

Personalized Nutrition for Gut Health

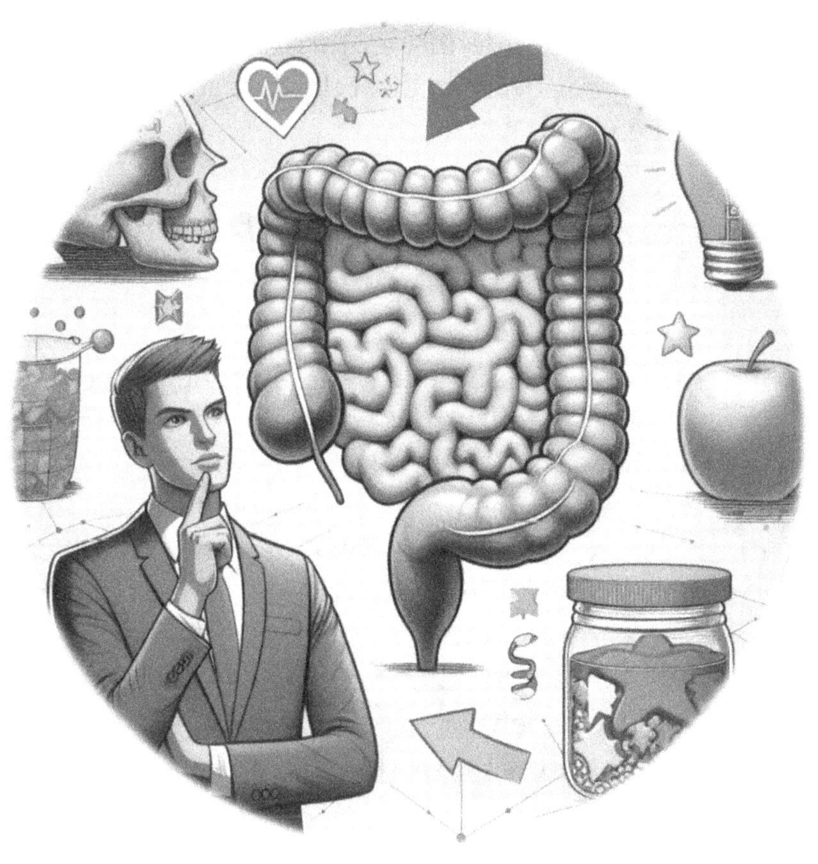

Gut health is not a one-size-fits-all concept. Each individual's microbiome is as unique as a fingerprint, influenced by factors such as genetics, diet, lifestyle, and environmental exposures. In this chapter, we'll explore the importance of recognizing individual differences in gut health, strategies for tracking and monitoring gut health, how to adjust your diet based on your personal gut health needs, the significance of working with a healthcare professional, using elimination diets to identify gut irritants, and building a sustainable gut-healthy lifestyle that supports long-term well-being.

Recognizing Individual Differences in Gut Health

While there are certain dietary and lifestyle factors that can promote overall gut health, it's essential to recognize that what works for one person may not work for another. Factors such as genetics, age, sex, medical history, and gut microbiome composition can all influence an individual's digestive function and tolerance to certain foods. Pay attention to your body's unique responses to different foods and lifestyle factors, and be open to experimenting with various approaches to find what works best for you.

How to Track and Monitor Gut Health

Tracking and monitoring your gut health can provide valuable insights into the factors that influence your digestive function and overall well-being. Keep a food and symptom journal to record what you eat and any symptoms or reactions you experience afterward. Look for patterns or correlations between specific foods or lifestyle factors and your digestive symptoms, such as bloating, gas, abdominal pain, or changes in bowel habits. Consider using digital health tools or apps to track your dietary intake, physical activity, sleep patterns, and stress levels to gain a comprehensive understanding of your gut health.

Adjusting Diet Based on Personal Gut Health Needs

Once you've identified patterns or triggers that affect your gut health, you can begin to make targeted adjustments to your diet and lifestyle to support optimal digestive function. Experiment with eliminating or reducing potential trigger foods such as gluten, dairy, refined sugars, artificial sweeteners, and processed foods to see if symptoms improve. Focus on incorporating whole, nutrient-dense foods such as fruits, vegetables, whole grains, lean proteins, and healthy fats to provide essential nutrients and support a balanced gut microbiome. Pay attention to portion sizes, meal timing, and meal composition to optimize digestion and prevent discomfort.

Importance of Working with a Healthcare Professional

While self-experimentation can be informative, it's essential to work with a qualified healthcare professional, such as a registered dietitian, nutritionist, or gastroenterologist, to develop a personalized approach to gut health. A healthcare professional can help interpret your symptoms, guide you through the process of elimination diets, and provide evidence-based recommendations tailored to your unique needs and preferences. They can also order diagnostic tests, such as stool analysis or food sensitivity testing, to identify underlying gut health issues and inform your treatment plan.

Using Elimination Diets to Identify Gut Irritants

Elimination diets involve temporarily removing certain foods or food groups from your diet and then systematically reintroducing them to identify potential triggers of digestive symptoms. Common elimination diets include the low FODMAP diet, which restricts fermentable carbohydrates that may contribute to gastrointestinal symptoms in some individuals, and the elimination-provocation diet, which involves removing suspected trigger foods and gradually reintroducing them while monitoring symptoms. Keep a detailed food and symptom journal during the elimination and reintroduction phases to track your body's responses and identify specific triggers.

Building a Sustainable Gut-Healthy Lifestyle

Creating a sustainable gut-healthy lifestyle involves more than just dietary changes—it's about adopting holistic habits that promote overall well-being and long-term digestive health. Focus on incorporating a diverse range of nutrient-dense foods, staying hydrated, managing stress, getting regular exercise, prioritizing sleep, and cultivating a supportive social network. Aim for balance, flexibility, and moderation in your approach to health, and be patient and compassionate with yourself as you navigate the journey toward optimal gut health.

Conclusion

Personalized nutrition plays a key role in supporting gut health and overall well-being. By recognizing individual differences in gut health, tracking and monitoring symptoms, adjusting your diet based on personal needs, working with healthcare professionals, using elimination diets to identify triggers, and building sustainable lifestyle habits, you can optimize your digestive function and promote long-term gut health. Remember that achieving optimal gut health is a journey that requires patience, experimentation, and ongoing self-discovery. Embrace the process, listen to your body, and prioritize self-care to nourish your unique microbiome and thrive from the inside out.

Chapter 15

Long-Term Gut Health Maintenance

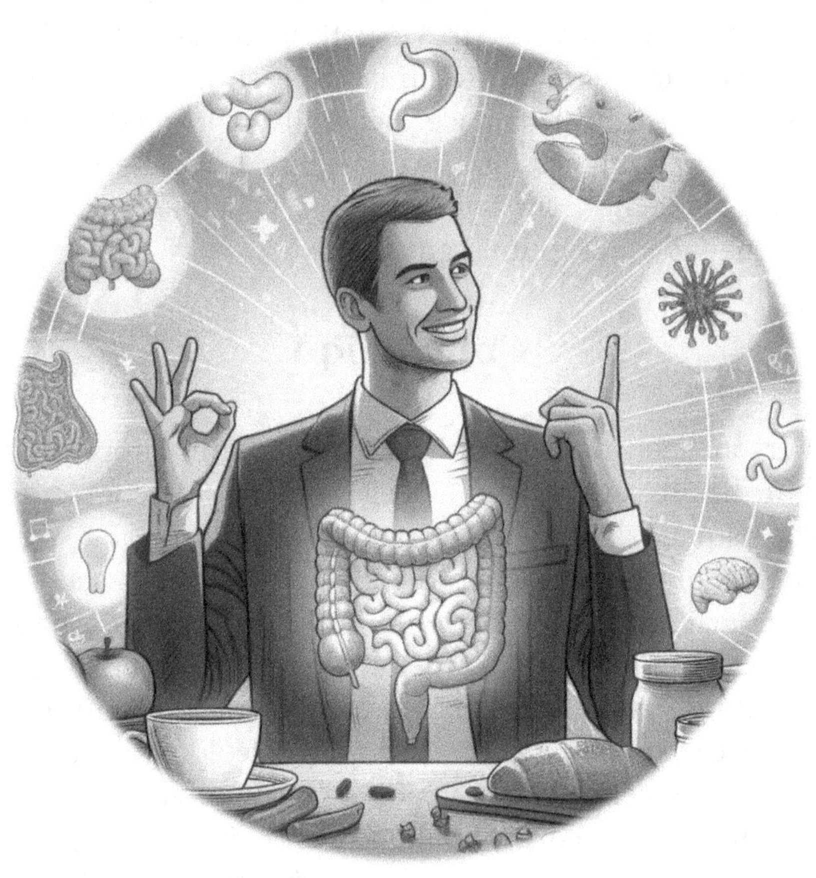

Maintaining gut health over the long term requires dedication, consistency, and a proactive approach to wellness. In this chapter, we'll delve deeper into strategies for sustaining gut health over time, emphasizing the importance of regular check-ins and adjustments, continuing education, building a supportive community, avoiding common pitfalls, staying motivated, and celebrating progress along the way. By prioritizing holistic well-being and nurturing a resilient gut microbiome, you can enjoy lasting vitality and thrive in your gut wellness journey.

Strategies for Maintaining Gut Health Over Time

Sustaining gut health isn't just about making short-term changes; it's about adopting sustainable lifestyle habits that support optimal digestive function and overall well-being. Here are some key strategies to consider:

Consistent Dietary Habits

Maintain a balanced and varied diet rich in whole, nutrient-dense foods that support gut health, including fruits, vegetables, whole grains, lean proteins, and healthy fats. Aim for consistency in your dietary habits, focusing on regular meal times, portion control, and mindful eating practices.

Regular Physical Activity

Incorporate regular physical activity into your routine to promote digestive motility, reduce stress, and support overall health. Choose activities that you enjoy and can sustain long term, whether it's walking, cycling, swimming, yoga, or strength training. Aim for at least 150 minutes of moderate-intensity exercise or 75 minutes of vigorous-intensity exercise per week, as recommended by health guidelines.

Stress Management Techniques

Implement stress management techniques such as mindfulness meditation, deep breathing exercises, yoga, or progressive muscle relaxation to reduce stress levels and support gut health. Prioritize self-care activities that promote relaxation and rejuvenation, such as spending time in nature, practicing gratitude, or engaging in creative hobbies.

Adequate Hydration

Stay hydrated by drinking plenty of water throughout the day to support digestive function and overall health. Aim to consume at least 8-10 cups of water per day, adjusting your fluid intake based on factors such as climate, physical activity level, and individual hydration needs.

Quality Sleep

Prioritize quality sleep to support gut health and overall well-being. Aim for 7-9 hours of uninterrupted sleep per night, creating a relaxing bedtime routine and optimizing your sleep environment for restorative rest. Practice good sleep hygiene habits, such as limiting screen time before bed, avoiding caffeine and alcohol close to bedtime, and maintaining a consistent sleep schedule.

Importance of Regular Check-Ins and Adjustments

Regular check-ins with yourself and healthcare professionals are crucial for monitoring gut health and making necessary adjustments to your wellness plan. Schedule periodic appointments with a registered dietitian, nutritionist, or gastroenterologist to assess your progress, discuss any changes in symptoms or dietary habits, and modify your treatment plan as needed. Be proactive in addressing emerging issues or concerns to prevent them from escalating into more significant problems down the line.

Continuing Education About Gut Health

Gut health is a dynamic and evolving field, with new research and insights emerging regularly. Stay informed about the latest developments in gut health by seeking out reputable sources of information, such as scientific journals, books, podcasts, and online resources. Attend educational seminars, workshops, or conferences to deepen your understanding of gut health and stay up-to-date on evidence-based practices and interventions.

Building a Supportive Community

Surround yourself with a supportive community of friends, family, healthcare professionals, and fellow gut health enthusiasts who share your values and goals. Join online or in-person support groups, forums, or social media communities where you can connect with others who are on a similar wellness journey. Share your experiences, ask questions, offer support and encouragement to fellow members, and celebrate each other's successes and milestones.

Avoiding Common Pitfalls and Staying Motivated

Maintaining gut health can be challenging at times, especially when faced with temptation, stress, or setbacks. Be mindful of common pitfalls such as relying on quick fixes or fad diets, neglecting self-care practices, or becoming overly fixated on symptoms or outcomes. Instead, focus on adopting sustainable habits that promote overall well-being and resilience.

Stay motivated by setting realistic goals, tracking your progress, celebrating small victories, and reminding yourself of the positive impact that gut health has on your life.

Celebrating Progress and Enjoying the Journey

Take time to celebrate your achievements and milestones along the gut health journey. Whether it's overcoming digestive challenges, adopting healthier habits, or experiencing improvements in symptoms, acknowledge and celebrate your progress. Treat yourself to small rewards or indulgences as a way of recognizing your hard work and dedication. Remember to enjoy the journey and appreciate the process of self-discovery and growth that comes with nurturing your gut health.

Conclusion

Maintaining long-term gut health is a journey that requires dedication, patience, and ongoing effort. By incorporating strategies for sustaining gut health over time, such as regular check-ins, continuing education, building a supportive community, avoiding common pitfalls, staying motivated, and celebrating progress, you can cultivate a resilient and vibrant gut microbiome that supports your overall well-being and vitality. Embrace the journey toward optimal gut health as an opportunity for growth, self-discovery, and empowerment, and remember that every step you take toward nurturing your gut is a step toward a healthier, happier life.

CONCLUSION

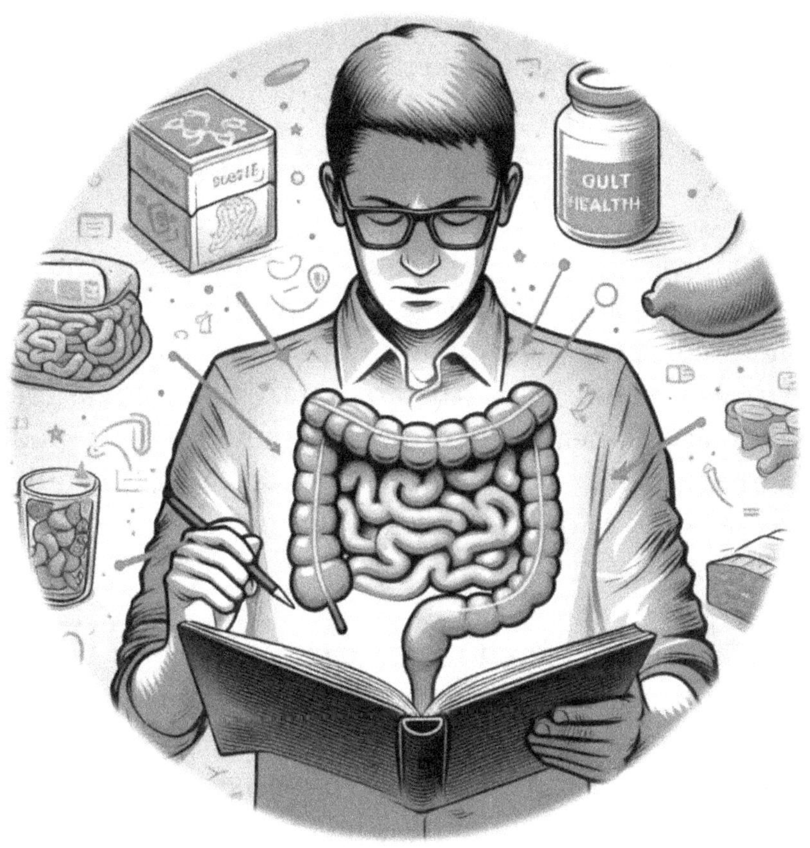

Congratulations on completing your journey toward a healthier gut! Throughout this book, we've delved deep into the intricate world of gut health, from unraveling the mysteries of the microbiome to implementing practical strategies for nurturing your digestive wellness. As you reflect on your experience and prepare to embark on the next phase of your wellness journey, let's take a moment to recap key insights, offer encouragement for the road ahead, emphasize the importance of patience and consistency, provide resources for further learning and support, offer final words of motivation and inspiration, and extend an invitation to connect and share experiences with fellow wellness seekers.

Recap of Key Points

Our journey began with a foundational understanding of gut health, exploring the vital role of the microbiome in digestion, immunity, and overall health. We examined how dietary and lifestyle factors influence gut health, identifying common signs of poor gut health and introducing the concept of gut-healthy recipes as a delicious way to support digestive wellness.

In Part 1, we explored the fundamentals of gut health, including the importance of the gut microbiome, the impact of dietary disruptors, the benefits of fiber intake, and the role of hydration in digestive function. We learned how to identify and avoid gut disruptors, boost fiber intake, and adopt an anti-inflammatory diet to support gut health.

Part 2 introduced advanced strategies and lifestyle tips for optimizing gut health, from harnessing the power of probiotics and prebiotics to managing stress and staying active. We discussed personalized nutrition for gut health, the significance of long-term maintenance, and strategies for avoiding common pitfalls and staying motivated on the wellness journey.

Encouragement to Take Actionable Steps

As you continue your journey toward optimal gut health, I encourage you to take actionable steps based on the insights and strategies you've gained from this book. Start by implementing small changes into your daily routine, such as incorporating more fiber-rich foods, hydrating regularly, and practicing stress management techniques. Remember that every step you take, no matter how small, brings you closer to vibrant health and well-being.

Importance of Patience and Consistency

Improving gut health is a journey that requires patience, consistency, and dedication. Be gentle with yourself and trust in the process of gradual progress. Celebrate the small victories along the way and learn from any setbacks or challenges you encounter. Stay committed to nurturing your gut health with consistent habits and positive lifestyle choices, knowing that your efforts will yield lasting benefits in the long run.

Resources for Further Learning and Support

As you continue to explore and deepen your understanding of gut health, consider seeking out additional resources for further learning and support. Look for reputable books, articles, podcasts, and online communities dedicated to gut health and holistic wellness. Connect with qualified healthcare professionals, such as registered dietitians or gastroenterologists, who can offer personalized guidance and support tailored to your individual needs.

Final Words of Motivation and Inspiration

As you navigate the twists and turns of your gut health journey, remember that you are not alone. Draw inspiration from the progress you've made and the transformations you've experienced along the way. Embrace each day as an opportunity to nourish and nurture your digestive wellness, knowing that your efforts are making a profound difference in your health and happiness. Stay resilient, stay focused, and stay hopeful, knowing that the path to vibrant gut health is paved with perseverance and positivity.

Invitation to Connect and Share Experiences

Your gut health journey is a unique and deeply personal experience, but it's also a journey that you don't have to navigate alone. I invite you to connect with others who share your passion for gut health and holistic wellness. Share your experiences, insights, and challenges with fellow wellness seekers, and offer support and encouragement along the way. Together, we can inspire and empower each other to thrive and flourish on our wellness journeys.

Thank you for embarking on this transformative journey toward a healthier gut. May you continue to nourish and nurture your digestive wellness with love, intention, and a sense of adventure. Here's to vibrant health, boundless vitality, and the joy of living life to the fullest. Cheers to your gut health journey!

ABOUT THE AUTHOR

Adeel Anjum is a visionary business leader with an illustrious career spanning over 20 years in strategic management and consulting. With a dynamic background that includes diverse industries such as sports retail, fashion retail, food retail, oil & gas, F&B, fitness & leisure, as well as technology & telecom retail, Adeel has amassed a wealth of experience and expertise in driving organizational success.

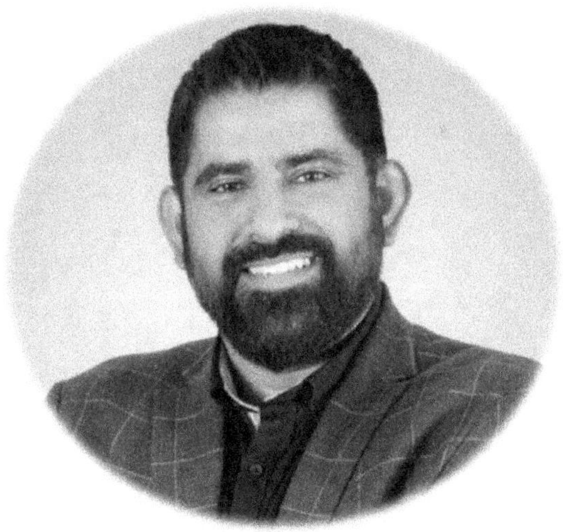

As a thought leader, Adeel Anjum stands at the forefront of shaping the business community through his pioneering work, insightful writings, and groundbreaking research. With a commitment to innovation and a deep understanding of Industry dynamics, Adeel Anjum inspires and guides fellow professionals, fostering a culture of continuous learning and strategic evolution within the business landscape.

Driven by a steadfast commitment to contribute to the business world, I am channeling my knowledge and experience into meaningful narratives within my books. My aim is to offer valuable insights, lessons, and strategies that empower individuals and organizations. Through the written word, I aspire to give back to the business community, sharing the wisdom gained on my journey and inspiring others to achieve their fullest potential and mindfulness.